BEGINNERS' GUIDE TO ESSENTIAL OILS

A Comprehensive Guide to Aromatherapy and Recipes for Natural Remedies

Robert Mauriello

TABLE OF CONTENTS

INTRODUCTION.. **6**

Definition and History..6

What Are Essential Oils?...........................6

History of Essential Oils..............................7

Extraction Methods...................................... 10

Overview of Different Types of Essential Oils.. 10

Overview of Different Types of Essential Oils. 13

Benefits of Essential Oils.................................. 18

Physical Health Benefits.......................18

Mental and Emotional Benefits.......................21

Uses in Daily Life...............................23

Chapter 1:... **26**

The Basics of Essential Oils.............................26

Understanding Essential Oils:............ 26

Chemical Composition.................................. 26

Volatility and Potency.................................... 28

Purity and Quality...29

How Essential Oils Work.............................32

Chapter 2:... **40**

Essential Oils and Safety................................. 40

General Safety Guidelines.............................. 40

Dilution and Carriers...................................... 42

Patch Testing...44

Safe Storage... 45

Specific Safety Considerations....................... 47

2. Children and Infants................................51

3. Pets..54

Common Mistakes and How to Avoid Them...57

Chapter 3:..**66**

Popular Essential Oils and Their Uses............66

Chapter 4:...**0**

Methods of Use...0

Aromatherapy...0

Inhalation Techniques..0

Topical Application...0

Compresses and Poultices...................................0

Skincare and Beauty..0

Internal Use...0

Supplements and Capsules..................................0

Chapter 5:...**0**

Creating Your Own Blends....................................0

Measuring and Recording Blends........................0

Blending for Specific Purposes...........................0

Relaxation and Stress Relief.................................0

Energy and Focus...0

Sleep and Insomnia..0

Pain and Inflammation...0

Skin Care and Beauty...0

Cleaning and Disinfecting.....................................0

Chapter 6:...**0**

Essential Oils for Health and Wellness.............0

Physical Health Applications...............................0

Immune System Support.......................................0

Respiratory Health...0

Mental and Emotional Wellness...........................0

Stress and Anxiety Relief...0

Mood Enhancement...0

Cognitive Function and Concentration...............0

Chronic Conditions and Long-term Use of
Essential Oils.. 0

Chronic Fatigue Syndrome............................... 0

Chapter 7:.. **0**

Essential Oils in Everyday Life..........................0

Natural Air Fresheners..0

Pest Control... 0

Beauty and Personal Care..................................0

DIY Skincare Recipes..0

Cooking and Food Preservation....................... 0

Chapter 8:.. **0**

Purchasing and Storing Essential Oils.............0

Storing Your Oils... 0

Chapter 9:.. **0**

The Science Behind Essential Oils................... 0

Phytochemistry of Essential Oils......................0

Research and Evidence.......................................0

Efficacy and Limitations:.................................... 0

Technological Advancements:............................0

CONCLUSION...**0**

Recap of Key Points..............................0

Understanding Essential Oils: Essential
oils are highly concentrated plant
extracts with unique properties. They
have a rich history and diverse uses,
ranging from physical and mental health
benefits to applications in beauty,
cleaning, and cooking.............................0

Encouragement for Further Exploration 0
APPENDICES...0
Glossary of Terms.. 0
Conversion Charts... 0

INTRODUCTION

Definition and History

What Are Essential Oils?

Essential oils are concentrated plant extracts that capture the natural scent, flavor, and beneficial properties of their source plants. They are called "essential" because they contain the "essence" of the plant's fragrance and its healing qualities. These oils are typically extracted from various parts of the plant, such as flowers, leaves, bark, roots, and peels, using methods like steam distillation or cold pressing.

To put it simply, when you crush a mint leaf between your fingers and inhale that strong, refreshing scent, you're experiencing the essential oil of mint in its natural form.

History of Essential Oils

The use of essential oils dates back thousands of years. Ancient civilizations recognized the powerful properties of these oils and incorporated them into their daily lives for various purposes, including medicinal, spiritual, and cosmetic.

1. **Ancient Egypt**: The Egyptians were among the first to utilize essential oils extensively. They used oils in their mummification processes, religious rituals, and for medicinal purposes. Oils like frankincense, myrrh, and cedarwood were particularly valued.
2. **China and India:** In China, essential oils have been used since ancient times for their medicinal properties. Chinese traditional medicine often incorporates these oils to treat various ailments.

Similarly, in India, essential oils play a crucial role in Ayurvedic medicine. The ancient texts of Ayurveda detail the use of oils like sandalwood, jasmine, and ginger for healing and balance.

3. **Greece and Rome:** The Greeks adopted knowledge from the Egyptians and expanded on it. Hippocrates, often referred to as the "father of medicine," used essential oils for their therapeutic benefits.

The Romans further popularized the use of essential oils in their daily lives, particularly for bathing and massage, valuing their aromatic and healing qualities.

4. **Middle Ages:** During the Middle Ages, essential oils were used throughout Europe for their medicinal properties. They were often the primary treatment for

many diseases and were also used in perfumes and cosmetics.

5. **Renaissance to Modern Times:** The Renaissance saw a revival in the use of essential oils, with notable figures like Paracelsus promoting their benefits. The scientific study of essential oils began to develop, leading to a better understanding of their properties and potential uses.

In modern times, essential oils have gained renewed popularity as people seek natural and holistic approaches to health and wellness. Today, they are used in aromatherapy, personal care products, household cleaning, and even as natural remedies.

Understanding the definition and history of essential oils helps us appreciate their value and versatility. These powerful plant extracts have been a part of human culture for millennia, and their benefits are still relevant today. Whether you're looking to improve your health, enhance your beauty routine, or simply enjoy the aromatic pleasure they offer, essential oils can be a wonderful addition to your life.

Extraction Methods

Overview of Different Types of Essential Oils

Essential oils are derived from plants through several extraction methods. Each method has its unique process and is chosen based on the type of plant material and the desired quality of the oil. Here are the most common extraction methods:

1.**Steam Distillation**: This is the most widely used method for extracting essential oils. It involves passing steam through the plant material, which causes the essential oils to evaporate. The steam containing the essential oils is then condensed back into liquid form and collected. The oil separates from the water and is skimmed off.

Example: Lavender oil, eucalyptus oil.

2. Cold Pressing: Also known as expression, this method is primarily used for citrus oils. The rinds of the fruit are mechanically pressed to release the essential oil. This process doesn't involve heat, preserving the oil's natural scent and properties.

Example: Lemon oil, orange oil.

3. Solvent Extraction: This method is used for delicate flowers and plants that don't yield much oil through steam distillation. Solvents like hexane or ethanol are used to dissolve the essential oil from the plant material. The solvent is then evaporated, leaving behind the concentrated oil.

Example: Jasmine oil, rose oil.

4. CO2 Extraction: This advanced method uses carbon dioxide under high pressure to extract essential oils. It's highly efficient and produces high-quality oils without the use of solvents. The CO2 is removed at the end, leaving a pure essential oil.

Example: Frankincense oil, ginger oil.

5. Maceration: In this method, plant material is soaked in a carrier oil to release its essential oils. The mixture is then heated and strained, resulting in an infused oil. This method is often used for making herbal oils rather than pure essential oils.

Example: Calendula oil, arnica oil.

6.Water Distillation: Similar to steam distillation, but the plant material is soaked in water rather than having steam passed through it. This method is less common but still used for certain plants.

Example: Rose water, orange blossom water.

Overview of Different Types of Essential Oils

Essential oils come from various parts of plants and have diverse properties and uses. Here's an overview of some popular types:

1.Lavender Oil:

Extraction Method: Steam distillation.

Uses: Known for its calming and relaxing properties, lavender oil is often used to reduce stress, improve sleep, and soothe skin irritations.

2. Peppermint Oil:

Extraction Method: Steam distillation.

Uses: This refreshing oil is used to alleviate headaches, improve digestion, and relieve muscle pain.

3. Tea Tree Oil:

Extraction Method: Steam distillation.

Uses: Famous for its antibacterial and antifungal properties, tea tree oil is commonly used to treat acne, dandruff, and minor cuts.

4. Eucalyptus Oil:

Extraction Method: Steam distillation.

Uses: Eucalyptus oil is often used to relieve respiratory issues, reduce inflammation, and act as a natural insect repellent.

5. Lemon Oil:

Extraction Method: Cold pressing.

Uses: This bright, uplifting oil is used to boost mood, support immune function, and clean surfaces.

6.Frankincense Oil:

Extraction Method: Steam distillation or CO_2 extraction.

Uses: Known for its grounding and spiritual properties, frankincense oil is used in meditation, skincare, and to reduce inflammation.

7. Rose Oil:

Extraction Method: Solvent extraction.

Uses: Valued for its rich, floral scent and skin-enhancing properties, rose oil is often used in perfumes and high-end skincare products.

8. Jasmine Oil:

Extraction Method: Solvent extraction.

Uses: This luxurious oil is known for its romantic scent and is used to uplift mood, reduce stress, and enhance skin elasticity.

9. Chamomile Oil:

Extraction Method: Steam distillation.

Uses: Chamomile oil is popular for its calming effects, making it useful for reducing anxiety, improving sleep, and soothing skin.

10. Ylang-Ylang Oil:

Extraction Method: Steam distillation.

Uses: With its sweet, floral aroma, ylang-ylang oil is used to reduce stress, lower blood pressure, and balance skin oils.

Each essential oil has its unique properties and benefits, making them versatile tools for natural health and wellness. By understanding the extraction methods and types of essential oils, you can choose the right oils for your needs and use them safely and effectively.

Benefits of Essential Oils

Essential oils are more than just pleasant scents; they offer a range of benefits for both physical health and mental well-being. Let's explore how these oils can enhance various aspects of our lives.

Physical Health Benefits

1. **Pain Relief:** Essential oils like peppermint, eucalyptus, and lavender are known for their analgesic properties. They can help alleviate headaches, muscle aches, and joint pain. For instance, applying a diluted mixture of peppermint oil to your temples can help reduce the intensity of a headache.

2. **Improved Digestion:** Oils such as ginger, peppermint, and fennel can support digestive health. They can relieve symptoms of indigestion, bloating, and gas. Ginger oil, for example, can be massaged onto the abdomen to soothe digestive discomfort.

3. **Enhanced Immune Function:** Essential oils like tea tree, eucalyptus, and lemon have antimicrobial properties that can help boost the immune system and fight off infections. Diffusing eucalyptus oil in your home can help purify the air and reduce the risk of respiratory infections.

4. **Respiratory Support:** Oils such as eucalyptus, peppermint, and rosemary can help clear the airways and improve breathing. Inhaling steam with a few drops of eucalyptus oil can provide relief from congestion and sinus issues.

5. **Skin Care:** Many essential oils have properties that benefit the skin. Tea tree oil is effective for acne, lavender oil can soothe irritated skin, and rose oil can hydrate and rejuvenate the skin. Adding a few drops of tea tree oil to your facial cleanser can help keep your skin clear.

6. **Anti-Inflammatory Effects:** Oils like frankincense, chamomile, and turmeric can reduce inflammation. These can be particularly helpful for conditions like arthritis. Massaging diluted chamomile oil onto inflamed joints can provide relief from pain and swelling.

Mental and Emotional Benefits

1. **Stress Relief:** Lavender, chamomile, and bergamot oils are known for their calming effects. They can help reduce stress and anxiety when inhaled or applied

topically. Diffusing lavender oil in your bedroom can create a serene environment conducive to relaxation.

2. **Mood Enhancement:** Citrus oils like lemon, orange, and grapefruit can uplift the mood and promote feelings of happiness. Inhaling the scent of these oils can help improve your overall sense of well-being.

3. **Improved Sleep:** Essential oils such as lavender, chamomile, and sandalwood can promote better sleep by creating a relaxing atmosphere. Applying a few drops of lavender oil to your pillow or using a diffuser in your bedroom can help you fall asleep more easily.

4. **Increased Focus and Concentration:** Oils like rosemary, peppermint, and lemon can enhance cognitive function and improve focus. Diffusing these

oils in your workspace can help you stay alert and productive.

5. **Emotional Balance:** Oils such as clary sage, ylang-ylang, and rose can help balance emotions and reduce feelings of sadness. Using these oils in a diffuser or as part of a massage can support emotional well-being.

Uses in Daily Life

1. **Aromatherapy**: Simply inhaling the scent of essential oils through a diffuser, spray, or even directly from the bottle can provide various benefits. Aromatherapy can be used to relax, energize, or create a particular mood in your living space.

2. **Massage**: Essential oils can be mixed with carrier oils (like coconut or jojoba oil) and used for massages. This allows the oils to be absorbed through the skin while providing the added benefit

of touch therapy. For example, a massage with lavender oil can help relieve muscle tension and stress.

3. **Skincare and Beauty**: Incorporating essential oils into your skincare routine can address various skin concerns. Adding a few drops of tea tree oil to your face wash can help with acne, while adding rose oil to your moisturizer can improve skin hydration.

4. **Household Cleaning:** Many essential oils have antimicrobial properties that make them effective natural cleaners. Lemon, tea tree, and eucalyptus oils can be used to make homemade cleaning solutions that disinfect and leave your home smelling fresh.

5. **Personal Care Products:** Essential oils can be added to homemade or store-bought products like shampoos, conditioners, and lotions. For

instance, adding a few drops of peppermint oil to your shampoo can invigorate your scalp and promote hair health.

6. **Cooking**: Certain essential oils, like lemon, peppermint, and ginger, can be used in cooking to add flavor and provide health benefits. Always use oils that are safe for ingestion and follow recommended guidelines.

7. **First Aid:** Essential oils can be part of your first aid kit. Lavender oil can be applied to minor cuts and burns for its soothing properties, while tea tree oil can be used on insect bites to reduce itching and swelling.

By understanding the benefits and versatile uses of essential oils, you can add these natural remedies into your daily routine to enhance your overall health and well-being. Whether you're trying to alleviate physical ailments, boost your mood, or simply enjoy the delightful scents, essential oils offer a wide range of possibilities.

Chapter 1:

The Basics of Essential Oils

Understanding Essential Oils:

To truly appreciate the power of essential oils, it's important to understand what they are and what makes them so special. In this chapter, we will look into the basics, covering their chemical composition, volatility and potency, and the importance of purity and quality.

Chemical Composition

Essential oils are complex mixtures of organic compounds produced by plants. These compounds include:

1. **Terpenes**: Terpenes are the largest and most varied class of compounds found in essential oils. They are responsible for the distinctive aromas of different oils and have various therapeutic

properties. For example, limonene (found in citrus oils) is uplifting and refreshing, while linalool (found in lavender) is calming and relaxing.

2. **Esters**: Esters often have fruity or floral scents and are known for their calming and anti-inflammatory properties. Lavender oil is rich in linalyl acetate, a type of ester that contributes to its soothing effects.

3. **Aldehydes**: These compounds typically have strong, pungent aromas and are known for their antimicrobial and anti-inflammatory properties. Cinnamaldehyde in cinnamon oil is a well-known example.

4. **Ketones**: Ketones can promote tissue regeneration and have mucolytic properties, which help in breaking down mucus. For instance, menthone is found in

peppermint oil and aids in respiratory health.

5. **Alcohols**: Alcohols in essential oils are known for their antimicrobial and antiseptic properties. Terpineol, found in tea tree oil, is a common example.

6. **Phenols**: Phenols are highly antiseptic and stimulating. Thymol, found in thyme oil, is a phenol known for its powerful antibacterial properties.

Each essential oil has a unique combination of these compounds, which determines its scent, properties, and uses.

Volatility and Potency

Essential oils are highly volatile, meaning they evaporate quickly when exposed to air. This volatility is what allows the aroma of the oils to be so noticeable and why they are so effective in aromatherapy. The small molecules in essential oils can quickly enter the air and be inhaled, allowing them to interact with the olfactory system and the brain.

The potency of essential oils is another key characteristic. Because they are highly concentrated extracts, even a small amount can have a significant effect. For instance, it can take hundreds of pounds of lavender flowers to produce just one pound of lavender essential oil. This concentration means that essential oils should always be used with care and respect, often requiring dilution before topical application.

Purity and Quality

The effectiveness and safety of essential oils depend greatly on their purity and quality. Here are some factors to consider:

1.Source: The quality of essential oils starts with the plants themselves. Factors like the species of the plant, the environment in which it's grown, and the harvesting methods all play a crucial role. High-quality essential oils come from plants that are grown in their native regions and are harvested at the right time.

2. **Extraction Method:** The method used to extract the oil can affect its purity. For instance, steam distillation and cold pressing are preferred for maintaining the integrity of the oils, while solvent extraction can sometimes leave residues that affect purity.

3. **Testing**: Reputable essential oil producers test their oils using methods like gas chromatography and mass spectrometry (GC/MS). These tests help ensure that the oils are pure, unadulterated, and contain the right balance of compounds.

4. **Certifications**: Look for oils that are certified organic or have other quality certifications. This can be an indicator that the oils have been produced without the use of pesticides or synthetic chemicals.

5. **Packaging**: Essential oils should be stored in dark glass bottles to protect them from light and degradation. Proper storage extends the shelf life and maintains the oil's efficacy.

6. **Reputation of Supplier:** Buying from reputable suppliers who are transparent about their sourcing and production processes can help ensure you are getting high-quality oils.

Understanding these basics helps you make informed decisions when selecting and using essential oils. By knowing what to look for in terms of chemical composition, volatility, potency, purity, and quality, you can ensure you are using oils that are both safe and effective.

How Essential Oils Work

Essential oils work in various ways to provide physical and mental benefits. Understanding these methods can help you use them more effectively and safely. Here's a detailed look at how essential oils interact with our bodies through absorption, inhalation, and even internal use.

1.Absorption Through the Skin:

When essential oils are applied to the skin, they don't just stay on the surface; they penetrate through the skin's layers and enter the bloodstream. This process can be enhanced by diluting the oils in carrier oils like coconut, jojoba, or almond oil, which also help prevent skin irritation from the concentrated essential oils.

<u>**Key Points:**</u>

A. **Massage and Skincare:**

Essential oils can be added to lotions, creams, and massage oils. During a massage, the combination of physical touch and the properties of the essential oils can help relax muscles, reduce pain, and improve circulation.

B. **Localized Application:**

For specific issues, such as muscle pain or skin conditions, applying essential oils directly to the affected area can provide targeted relief. For example, applying tea tree oil (diluted) to acne can help reduce inflammation and kill bacteria.

C. Foot Soaks and Baths:

Adding essential oils to bath water or a foot soak allows the oils to be absorbed over a larger area, providing overall relaxation and soothing sore muscles. A few drops of lavender oil in a warm bath can help promote relaxation and improve sleep.

The skin's ability to absorb essential oils means they can be used effectively for both localized treatment and systemic effects.

2. Inhalation and Olfactory System

Inhalation is one of the most popular ways to use essential oils, primarily because of its immediate impact on the brain and emotions. When you inhale essential oils, the molecules travel through the nose and stimulate the olfactory system, which is directly linked to the brain's limbic system, responsible for emotions, behavior, and memory.

Key Points:

A. Diffusers: Using an essential oil diffuser disperses the oil molecules into the air, allowing you to inhale them over time. This method is great for creating a specific atmosphere, such as calming or energizing your home or workspace. For instance, diffusing eucalyptus oil can help clear the airways and improve breathing.

B. **Direct Inhalation:** You can inhale essential oils directly from the bottle or by placing a few drops on a tissue or cotton ball. This method is useful for quick relief of symptoms like stress or nausea. Inhaling peppermint oil can help alleviate headaches and improve focus.

C. **Steam Inhalation:** Adding a few drops of essential oil to a bowl of hot water and inhaling the steam can provide therapeutic benefits, especially for respiratory issues. Covering your head with a towel and breathing in the steam infused with tea tree or eucalyptus oil can help clear nasal congestion.

The direct route from the nose to the brain means that inhaling essential oils can quickly affect mood, stress levels, and even cognitive function.

3. Internal Use (Controversies and Safety)

Using essential oils internally is a more controversial topic. While some practitioners and brands advocate for the internal use of certain essential oils, others caution against it due to potential risks.

<u>Key Points:</u>

A. **Potential Benefits:** Some essential oils can be ingested to aid digestion, support the immune system, or provide other health benefits. For example, adding a drop of lemon oil to water can act as a detoxifying agent and support digestion.

B. **Safety Concerns**: Essential oils are highly concentrated and can be toxic if used improperly. Not all essential oils are safe for internal use, and those that are should be used with great caution. It's crucial to ensure the oil is pure and labeled as safe for ingestion.

C. **Dosage and Dilution:** When using essential oils internally, they must be properly diluted to avoid irritation or toxicity. Even safe oils should be used sparingly. For instance, a single drop of peppermint oil can be added to a large amount of water or food.

D. **Consulting Professionals:** Before using essential oils internally, it's advisable to consult with a healthcare professional, especially if you have existing health conditions or are taking other medications. Professionals can provide guidance on safe usage and appropriate dosages.

Examples of Internal Use:

1. **Peppermint Oil**: Known to support digestion, it can be taken in very small amounts to relieve digestive discomfort.
2. **Lemon Oil**: Often used for its detoxifying properties, a drop can be added to water.
3. **Oregano Oil**: Sometimes used as a natural antibiotic, but must be heavily diluted and used with caution.

While internal use of essential oils can offer benefits, it's essential to prioritize safety and seek professional advice to avoid potential health risks.

By understanding these different methods of using essential oils—through the skin, inhalation, and internal use—you can make more informed choices and maximize the benefits while minimizing the risks. Essential oils can be a powerful tool for improving health and well-being when used correctly.

Chapter 2:

Essential Oils and Safety

Essential oils can offer many health benefits, but they must be used safely to avoid adverse effects. This chapter will guide you through general safety guidelines, proper dilution and carrier oils, patch testing, and safe storage practices.

General Safety Guidelines

1. **Know Your Oils:** Not all essential oils are created equal. Some are safe for most people, while others can be harmful if not used correctly. Educate yourself about the specific oils you plan to use, paying attention to any potential risks or contraindications.

2. **Use Pure Oils:** Always use high-quality, pure essential oils. Check for reputable brands that provide

information about the sourcing and testing of their products. Avoid oils with synthetic additives or fillers, which can cause skin irritation and reduce effectiveness.

3. Consult with a Professional: If you're new to essential oils or have existing health conditions, it's a good idea to consult with a healthcare professional or a certified aromatherapist. They can provide personalized advice and help you avoid potential interactions with medications or health issues.

4. Avoid Sensitive Areas: Never apply essential oils to sensitive areas such as the eyes, ears, mucous membranes, or broken skin. If an oil accidentally gets into your eyes, rinse immediately with a carrier oil (not water) and seek medical advice if necessary.

5. Start Slowly:

Begin with small amounts and see how your body reacts before increasing the dosage. This helps you identify any sensitivities or allergies early on.

6. Keep Away from Children and Pets: Essential oils can be particularly potent for children and pets. Always store oils out of their reach and use child-safe and pet-safe essential oils in lower dilutions when necessary.

Dilution and Carriers

Essential oils are highly concentrated and should almost always be diluted before use. Carrier oils are used to dilute essential oils, making them safe for topical application.

1. Why Dilute? Diluting essential oils helps prevent skin irritation, sensitization, and other adverse reactions. It also helps the essential oil spread more easily over the skin, enhancing its absorption.

2. Common Carrier Oils:

A. **Coconut Oil:** Moisturizing and lightweight, great for skin and hair.
B. **Jojoba Oil:** Closely resembles the skin's natural oils, making it excellent for all skin types.
C. **Sweet Almond Oil**: Rich in vitamins, suitable for dry and sensitive skin.
D. **Olive Oil**: Nourishing and readily available, though heavier than some other carriers.
E. **Grapeseed Oil**: Lightweight and quickly absorbed, ideal for massage oils.

3. Dilution Guidelines:

For adults, a common dilution ratio is 2-3 drops of essential oil per teaspoon (5 ml) of carrier oil (about a 2-3%

dilution). For children, elderly individuals, or those with sensitive skin, use a lower dilution of 1 drop per teaspoon (1% dilution).

For facial applications, use a very low dilution, such as 0.5% to 1%.

Patch Testing

Before using a new essential oil, it's important to perform a patch test to check for any allergic reactions or sensitivities.

1. **How to perform Patch Test:**

- Dilute the essential oil in a carrier oil (using a 1% dilution).
- Apply a small amount of the diluted oil to a patch of skin on your inner forearm.
- Cover the area with a bandage and leave it for 24 hours.

- Check for any redness, itching, or irritation. If you experience any adverse reactions, do not use the oil on your skin.

2. **Interpreting Results:**

- If there is no reaction after 24 hours, the oil is likely safe for use on your skin.
- If you experience any discomfort, redness, or swelling, avoid using that particular oil and consider consulting a healthcare professional.

Safe Storage

Proper storage of essential oils is crucial to maintaining their potency and extending their shelf life.

1. **Use Dark Glass Bottles:** Store essential oils in dark amber or cobalt blue glass bottles. These help protect the

oils from light, which can degrade their quality over time.

2. **Keep Away from Heat and Light:**

Store your oils in a cool, dark place, such as a cabinet or drawer. Avoid placing them near windows, heaters, or other sources of heat and light.

3. **Tightly Seal Bottles:** Ensure that the bottles are tightly sealed to prevent oxidation and evaporation. This helps preserve the oils' aromatic and therapeutic properties.

4. **Label Your Oils:** Clearly label each bottle with the oil's name, extraction date, and any other relevant information. This helps you keep track of their age and ensures you use them within their optimal time frame.

5. **Check Expiration Dates:**

Essential oils have varying shelf lives, typically ranging from 1 to 3 years.

Citrus oils tend to have shorter shelf lives, while oils like patchouli and sandalwood can last much longer. Regularly check your oils for any changes in scent, color, or consistency, which can indicate that they have degraded.

By following these safety guidelines, you can enjoy the many benefits of essential oils while minimizing the risk of adverse reactions. Safe practices, such as proper dilution, patch testing, and mindful storage, ensure that your experience with essential oils is both effective and enjoyable.

Specific Safety Considerations

Essential oils are powerful natural remedies, but certain groups—like pregnant and breastfeeding women, children and infants, and pets—require special safety precautions. This section will explore how to use essential oils safely for these vulnerable groups.

1.Pregnant and Breastfeeding Women: Pregnancy and breastfeeding are times when safety is paramount. Essential oils can be beneficial, but they must be used cautiously to avoid any potential risks to the mother and baby.

<u>**Key Considerations**</u>:

A.Consult a Healthcare Professional: Always talk to your doctor or a certified aromatherapist before using essential oils during pregnancy or while breastfeeding. They can provide personalized advice based on your specific situation.

B. Avoid Certain Oils: Some essential oils should be avoided during pregnancy due to their potential to stimulate contractions or cause other adverse effects. Oils to avoid include:

- **Clary Sage:** Can induce contractions.

- **Cinnamon**: May cause skin irritation and uterine contractions.
- **Rosemary**: Linked to increased blood pressure and uterine contractions.
- **Jasmine**: Can trigger contractions.
- **Sage**: May cause uterine contractions.

C. **Safe Oils for Pregnancy:** Many essential oils are considered safe for use during pregnancy when properly diluted. These include:

- **Lavender**: Helps with relaxation and sleep.
- **Chamomile**: Soothes anxiety and promotes relaxation.
- **Ylang-Ylang**: Calming and mood-lifting.
- **Frankincense**: Supports emotional well-being and reduces stress.

D. Proper Dilution: Use a lower dilution rate of 1% (1 drop of essential oil per teaspoon of carrier oil) to minimize the risk of skin irritation and other adverse effects.

E. Topical Use and Diffusion:

Topical application (properly diluted) and diffusion are generally safer methods. Avoid internal use of essential oils during pregnancy and breastfeeding.

F. Breastfeeding Considerations: Be cautious with oils applied to the chest or near the baby's mouth. Oils like peppermint can reduce milk supply, so avoid using them in large amounts.

2. Children and Infants

Children and infants have more sensitive skin and developing systems, so essential oils must be used with extra care.

<u>**Key Considerations:**</u>

A. Age Appropriateness: Avoid using essential oils on infants under 3 months old. For older infants and young children, use only mild oils and at very low dilutions.

B. Safe Oils for Children: Some essential oils are safer for use with children, including:

- **Lavender**: Gentle and calming, suitable for promoting sleep.
- **Chamomile**: Soothes and calms both skin and mood.
- **Frankincense**: Supports respiratory health and relaxation.
- **Tea Tree (Melaleuca)**: Effective for minor cuts and scrapes, but must be properly diluted.

C. Proper Dilution: Use a very low dilution for children:

- **Infants (3 months to 2 years):** 0.25% dilution (1 drop per 4 teaspoons of carrier oil).
- **Children (2 to 6 years):** 1% dilution (1 drop per teaspoon of carrier oil).
- **Children (6 to 12 years):** 1-2% dilution (1-2 drops per teaspoon of carrier oil).

D. Patch Testing: Always perform a patch test before using a new essential oil on a child's skin to check for any allergic reactions or sensitivities.

E. Avoid Certain Oils: Some oils are not safe for young children and should be avoided, including:

- **Peppermint:** Can cause respiratory issues in young children.

- **Eucalyptus**: Contains compounds that can be harmful to infants and young children.
- **Wintergreen**: Highly toxic if ingested and can cause severe reactions.

F. **Inhalation**: Use diffusers in well-ventilated areas and for short periods (30 minutes at a time) to ensure the child's safety and comfort.

3. Pets

Pets, particularly cats and dogs, are sensitive to essential oils. What might be safe for humans can be harmful or even toxic to animals.

<u>Key Considerations:</u>

A. **Species Sensitivity:** Cats are particularly sensitive to essential oils due to their unique liver metabolism.

Avoid using essential oils around cats unless advised by a veterinarian.

Dogs can tolerate some essential oils, but caution is still necessary. Birds and other small animals are highly sensitive and should generally not be exposed to essential oils.

B. **Safe Oils for Dogs:** Some oils can be used safely with dogs, but always in very low dilutions and under professional guidance. Safe oils may include:

- **Lavender**: Calming and soothing.
- **Chamomile**: Gentle and anti-inflammatory.
- **Frankincense**: Supports overall health and well-being.

C. **Avoid Certain Oils:** Many essential oils are toxic to pets, including:

- **Tea Tree (Melaleuca):** Toxic to both cats and dogs if ingested or applied in large amounts.
- **Pennyroyal**: Highly toxic to pets.
- **Wintergreen**: Contains methyl salicylate, which is toxic to pets.
- **Citrus Oils (lemon, orange, lime):** Can cause vomiting and other adverse reactions in pets.

D. Proper Dilution and Application: Always dilute essential oils heavily before using them around pets. A safe dilution for pets is usually around 0.25% (1 drop per 4 teaspoons of carrier oil).

Apply oils to areas where the pet cannot lick them, such as the back of the neck.

E. Inhalation Safety: If using a diffuser, ensure the room is well-ventilated and the pet can leave the area if they choose. Avoid continuous diffusion and opt for intermittent use instead.

F. Consult with a Veterinarian: Always consult with a veterinarian knowledgeable about essential oils before using them around pets. They can provide specific advice based on your pet's health and needs.

By understanding and following these specific safety considerations, you can safely incorporate essential oils into your life while protecting the well-being of pregnant and breastfeeding women, children, and pets. Proper usage ensures that you and your loved ones can enjoy the benefits of essential oils without unnecessary risks.

Common Mistakes and How to Avoid Them

Essential oils can be incredibly beneficial, but it's easy to make mistakes if you're not careful. Understanding common errors and how to avoid them can help you use essential oils safely and effectively. This section will cover overuse and misuse, combining essential oils with medications, and recognizing adverse reactions.

Overuse and Misuse

1. Using Too Much Oil: Essential oils are potent, and using too much can lead to adverse effects like skin irritation, headaches, or nausea.

How to Avoid:

Dilution: Always dilute essential oils with a carrier oil. A general rule is to use a 2-3% dilution for adults (2-3 drops of essential oil per teaspoon of carrier oil). For children, elderly individuals, or those with sensitive skin, use a lower dilution (1% or less).

Start Small: Begin with a small amount and gradually increase if needed. For diffusers, 3-5 drops are usually sufficient.

2. Incorrect Application: Applying essential oils directly to the skin without proper dilution can cause burns, rashes, or other irritations.

How to Avoid:

Follow Guidelines: Always follow recommended dilution guidelines and usage instructions.

Sensitive Areas: Avoid applying oils to sensitive areas such as the eyes, ears, and mucous membranes.

3. Inadequate Knowledge: Using essential oils without proper knowledge can lead to misuse, such as ingesting oils that are not safe for internal use.

How to Avoid:

Educate Yourself: Learn about each oil's properties and safe uses before applying them. Consult reputable sources or professionals.

Read Labels: Pay attention to product labels and manufacturer instructions. Some oils are safe for certain applications while others are not.

Combining with Medications

1. Potential Interactions:

Essential oils can interact with medications, potentially altering their effects or causing side effects.

How to Avoid:

Consult a Professional: Before using essential oils, especially if you're on medication, consult with a healthcare provider or a certified aromatherapist.

Be Aware of Contraindications: Some oils, such as grapefruit oil, can affect how certain medications are metabolized.

2. Avoiding Specific Oils:

Certain essential oils should be avoided if you have specific health conditions or are taking particular medications.

How to Avoid:

Research: Investigate any contraindications for essential oils you intend to use. For example, if you are taking blood thinners, avoid oils like wintergreen, which can have blood-thinning effects.

3. Monitoring Effects:

If you combine essential oils with medications, monitor your body's response carefully.

How to Avoid:

Keep a Journal: Track your essential oil use and note any changes in your health or medication efficacy. This can help identify any adverse interactions.

Immediate Action: If you notice any negative reactions, stop using the essential oil immediately and consult a healthcare professional.

Recognizing Adverse Reactions

1. Skin Reactions:

Redness, itching, or burning sensations can indicate an adverse skin reaction.

<u>**How to Avoid:**</u>

Patch Testing: Before using a new essential oil, perform a patch test. Dilute the oil and apply a small amount to a patch of skin on your forearm. Wait 24 hours to see if there is any reaction.

Proper Dilution: Always dilute essential oils adequately before applying them to your skin.

2. Respiratory Issues: Some people may experience respiratory problems such as coughing, wheezing, or shortness of breath when using essential oils.

How to Avoid:

Use in Well-Ventilated Areas: When diffusing essential oils, ensure the area is well-ventilated.

Avoid Direct Inhalation: If you have a history of respiratory issues, avoid direct inhalation and consult a healthcare professional before use.

3. Systemic Reactions:

Nausea, dizziness, or headaches can indicate that your body is reacting adversely to essential oils.

How to Avoid:

Start Slowly: Begin with small amounts to see how your body reacts.

Recognize Symptoms: Be aware of any unusual symptoms after using essential oils. If you experience any adverse effects, discontinue use and seek medical advice if necessary.

4. Allergic Reactions:

In rare cases, essential oils can cause severe allergic reactions, such as difficulty breathing or swelling.

How to Avoid:

Know Your Allergies: Be aware of any known allergies to plants or plant extracts. Avoid oils from those plants.

Seek Immediate Help: If you experience severe allergic reactions, seek medical attention immediately.

By understanding these common mistakes and how to avoid them, you can use essential oils safely and effectively. Proper education, cautious application, and awareness of potential interactions and reactions are key to enjoying the benefits of essential oils while minimizing risks.

Chapter 3:

Popular Essential Oils and Their Uses

Essential oils each have unique properties and benefits. Here, we'll cover the top 20 essential oils for beginners, providing detailed profiles including their botanical names, main properties, uses and benefits, and blending tips.

1.Lavender *(Lavandula angustifolia)*

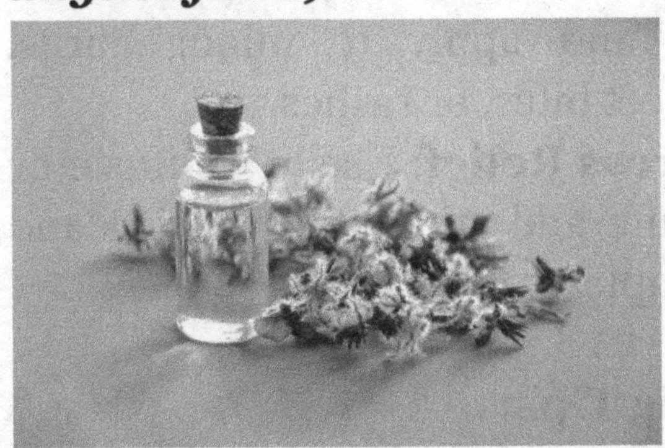

Botanical Name: *Lavandula angustifolia*

Main Properties:

- **Calming**: Promotes relaxation and helps reduce anxiety.
- **Antiseptic**: Helps cleanse and heal minor cuts and scrapes.
- **Anti-inflammatory**: Soothes skin irritations and reduces redness.

Uses and Benefits:

- **Relaxation and Sleep**: Add a few drops to your pillow or diffuse before bedtime to promote restful sleep.
- **Skin Care**: Dilute with a carrier oil and apply to minor burns, insect bites, or rashes.
- **Stress Relief**: Use in a diffuser or dilute and apply to the wrists and temples.

Blending Tips:

Blends well with citrus oils (lemon, orange), florals (rose, geranium), and herbaceous oils (rosemary, clary sage).

2. Peppermint (*Mentha piperita*)

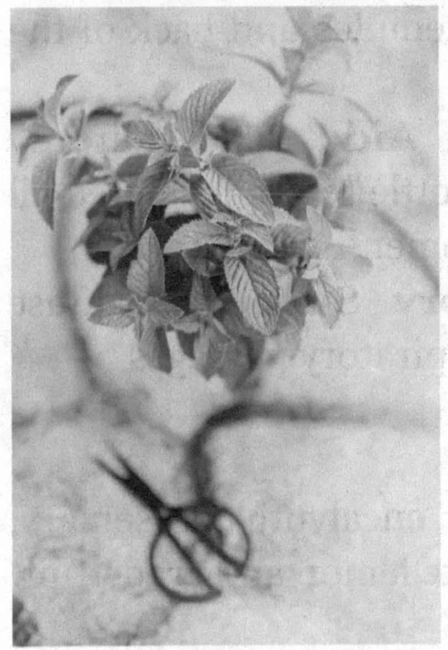

Botanical Name: *Mentha piperita*

Main Properties:

- **Cooling**: Provides a refreshing and cooling sensation.
- **Energizing**: Stimulates the mind and enhances focus.

- **Antimicrobial**: Fights bacteria and viruses.

Uses and Benefits:
- **Headache Relief**: Apply diluted oil to the temples and back of the neck.
- **Digestive Aid**: Inhale directly from the bottle or apply diluted oil to the abdomen.
- **Respiratory Support**: Diffuse to clear respiratory passages

Blending Tips:
Pairs well with eucalyptus, rosemary, and citrus oils like lemon and grapefruit.

3. Tea Tree (*Melaleuca alternifolia*)

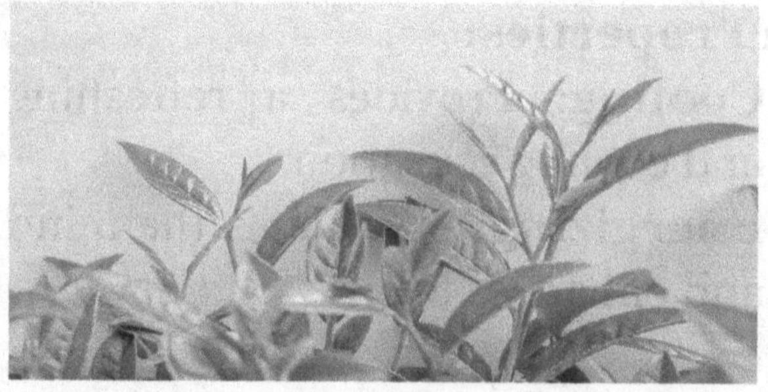

Botanical Name: *Melaleuca alternifolia*

Main Properties:
- **Antibacterial**: Fights bacterial infections.
- **Antifungal**: Effective against fungi like athlete's foot.
- **Antiseptic**: Cleanses wounds and prevents infection.

Uses and Benefits:
- **Acne Treatment:** Apply diluted oil to acne-prone areas to reduce breakouts.
- **Skin Infections**: Use on minor cuts and scrapes to prevent infection.
- **Home Cleaning**: Add to home-made cleaning products for its disinfectant properties.

Blending Tips:

Blends well with lavender, peppermint, eucalyptus, and lemon for enhanced antimicrobial effects.

4. Eucalyptus (*Eucalyptus globulus*)

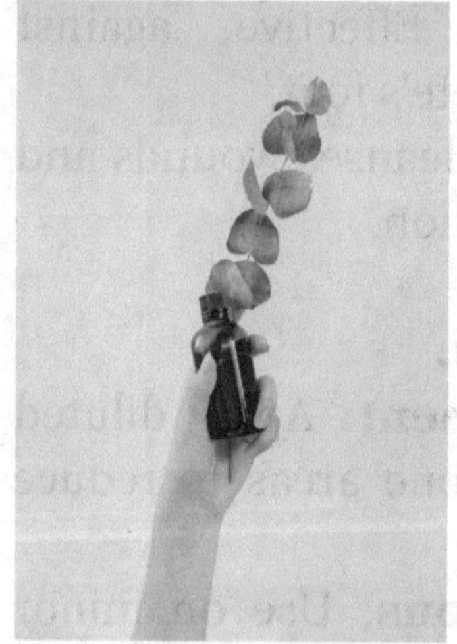

Botanical Name: *Eucalyptus globulus*

Main Properties:
- **Decongestant**: Clears nasal passages.
- **Antiviral**: Fights viral infections.
- **Anti-inflammatory**: Reduces inflammation.

Uses and Benefits:

- **Respiratory Health**: Diffuse to ease breathing during colds and flu.
- **Muscle Pain Relief**: Apply diluted oil to sore muscles.
- **Insect Repellent**: Use in a spray to repel insects.

Blending Tips:

Mix with tea tree, peppermint, rosemary, and lemon for respiratory and cleaning blends.

5. Lemon (*Citrus limon*)

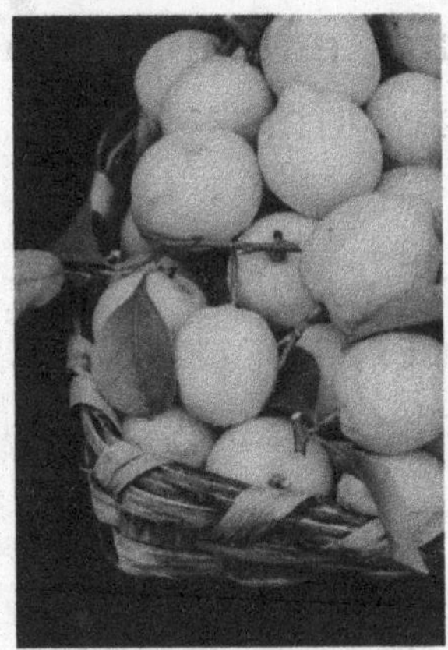

Botanical Name: *Citrus limon*

Main Properties:

- **Uplifting**: Enhances mood and energy.
- **Antiseptic**: Cleanses and disinfects.
- **Detoxifying**: Supports the body's detox processes.

Uses and Benefits:

- **Mood Booster:** Diffuse to uplift and energize.
- **Cleaning**: Add to cleaning solutions for its antibacterial properties.
- **Skin Care**: Dilute and apply to brighten and clarify skin.

Blending Tips:
Blends well with lavender, peppermint, eucalyptus, and other citrus oils.

6. Frankincense   (*Boswellia carteri*)

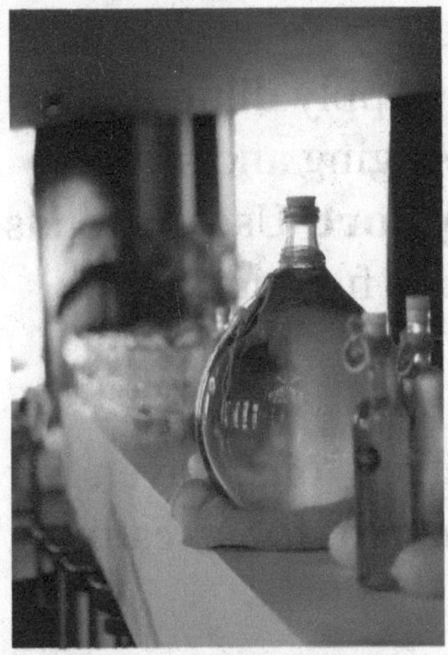

Botanical Name: *Boswellia carteri*

Main Properties:
- **Grounding**: Promotes relaxation and meditation.
- **Anti-inflammatory**: Reduces inflammation.
- **Immune-boosting**: Supports immune health.

Uses and Benefits:

- **Meditation Aid**: Diffuse during meditation or prayer for a grounding effect.
- **Skin Health**: Apply diluted oil to reduce signs of aging and scars.
- **Immune Support**: Use in blends to boost immune function.

Blending Tips:
Pairs well with citrus oils, lavender, sandalwood, and myrrh for a calming blend.

7. **Chamomile (*Matricaria chamomilla* or *Chamaemelum nobile*)**

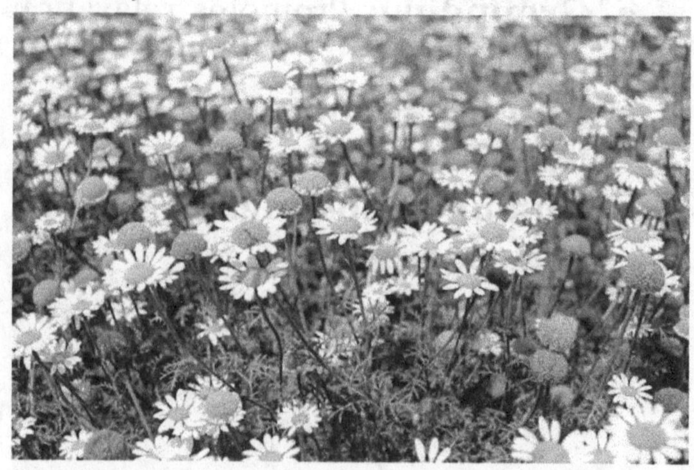

Botanical Name: *Matricaria chamomilla* (German chamomile) or *Chamaemelum nobile* (Roman chamomile)

Main Properties:
- **Calming**: Reduces anxiety and promotes relaxation.
- **Anti-inflammatory**: Soothes skin and reduces redness.
- **Antispasmodic**: Eases muscle spasms and cramps.

Uses and Benefits:
- **Stress Relief**: Diffuse or apply diluted oil to reduce anxiety.
- **Skin Care**: Use in skincare routines to soothe and heal skin.
- **Digestive Health**: Apply diluted oil to the abdomen to ease digestive discomfort.

Blending Tips:
Blends well with lavender, rose, geranium, and ylang-ylang.

8. Rose (*Rosa damascena*)

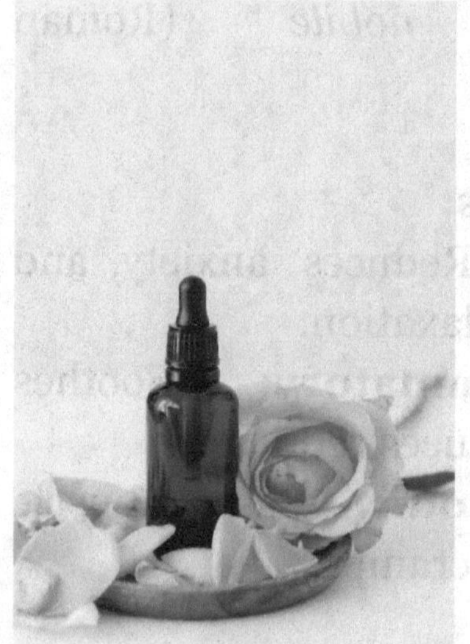

Botanical Name: *Rosa damascena*

Main Properties:

- **Antidepressant**: Enhances mood and reduces stress.
- **Astringent**: Tightens and tones skin.
- **Anti-inflammatory**: Reduces skin redness and irritation.

Uses and Benefits:

- **Emotional Well-being**: Diffuse to uplift and soothe emotions.
- **Skin Care**: Apply diluted oil to improve skin tone and texture.
- **Menstrual Relief**: Use in blends to ease menstrual discomfort.

Blending Tips:
Pairs beautifully with lavender, sandalwood, geranium, and jasmine.

9. Ylang-Ylang (*Cananga odorata*)

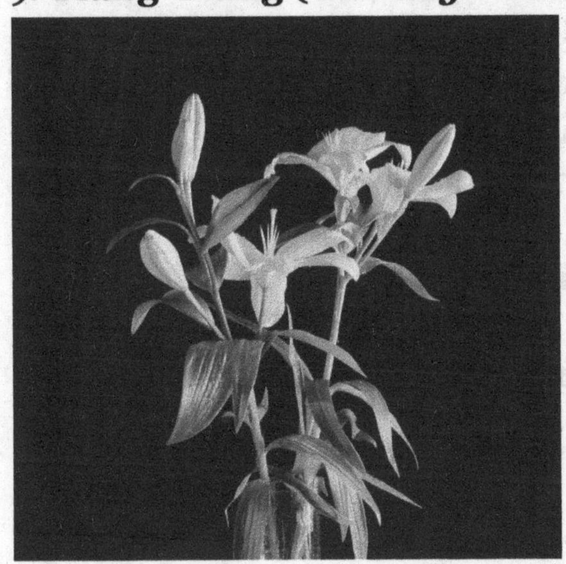

Botanical Name: *Cananga odorata*

Main Properties:

- **Sedative**: Promotes relaxation and reduces anxiety.
- **Antidepressant**: Uplifts mood and soothes emotions.
- **Antiseptic**: Cleanses and heals minor wounds.

Uses and Benefits:

- **Stress Relief:** Diffuse or apply diluted oil to reduce stress and promote relaxation.
- **Skin Care:** Use in skincare routines to balance oil production.
- **Aphrodisiac**: Diffuse to enhance romantic moods.

Blending Tips:

Blends well with citrus oils, lavender, and sandalwood for a soothing blend.

10. Clary Sage (*Salvia sclarea*)

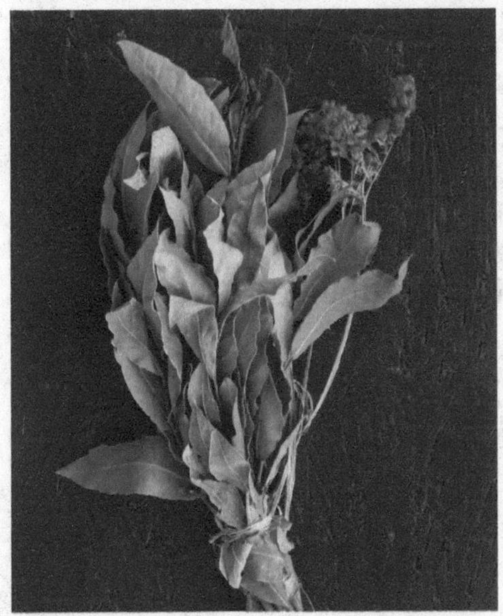

Botanical Name: *Salvia sclarea*

Main Properties:

- **Hormone-balancing**: Regulates hormonal fluctuations.
- **Antidepressant**: Uplifts mood and reduces stress.
- **Antispasmodic**: Eases muscle spasms and menstrual cramps.

Uses and Benefits:

- **Menstrual Relief:** Apply diluted oil to the abdomen to ease cramps.
- **Stress Reduction**: Diffuse or apply diluted oil to reduce anxiety and stress.
- **Sleep Aid**: Use in blends to promote restful sleep.

Blending Tips:
Mix with lavender, chamomile, and ylang-ylang for hormonal support and relaxation.

11.   Geranium   (*Pelargonium graveolens*)

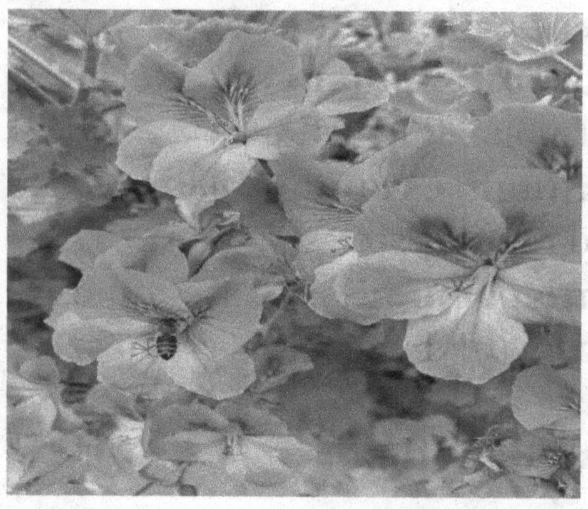

Botanical Name: *Pelargonium graveolens*

Main Properties:
- **Balancing**: Regulates skin and emotional balance.
- **Antibacterial**: Fights bacterial infections.
- **Anti-inflammatory**: Reduces inflammation and soothes skin.

Uses and Benefits:
- **Skin Care**: Apply diluted oil to balance oily or dry skin.
- **Emotional Balance**: Diffuse to promote emotional well-being.
- **Anti-inflammatory**: Use in blends to reduce inflammation and soothe skin irritations.

Blending Tips:
Blends well with lavender, clary sage, and rose for skincare and emotional balance.

12. Bergamot (*Citrus bergamia*)

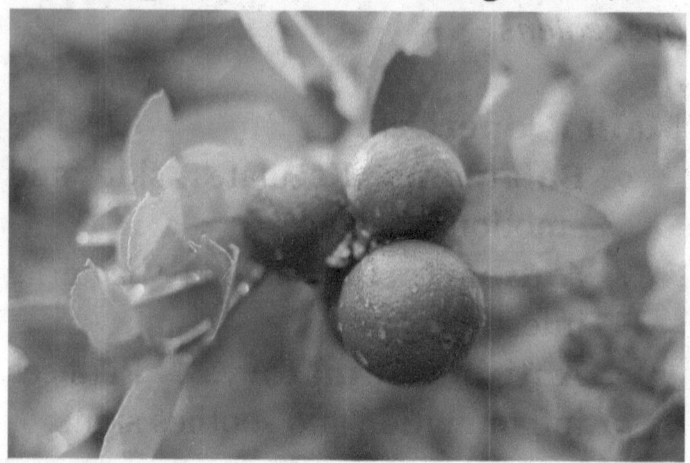

Botanical Name: *Citrus bergamia*

Main Properties:

- **Uplifting**: Enhances mood and reduces stress.
- **Antidepressant**: Boosts emotional well-being.
- **Antiseptic**: Cleanses and purifies skin.

Uses and Benefits:

- **Mood Enhancer:** Diffuse to uplift and reduce anxiety.
- **Skin Care**: Apply diluted oil to cleanse and purify skin.

- **Digestive Health**: Use in blends to support digestion.

Blending Tips:
Blends beautifully with lavender, ylang-ylang, and other citrus oils for a refreshing blend.

13. Sandalwood (*Santalum album*)

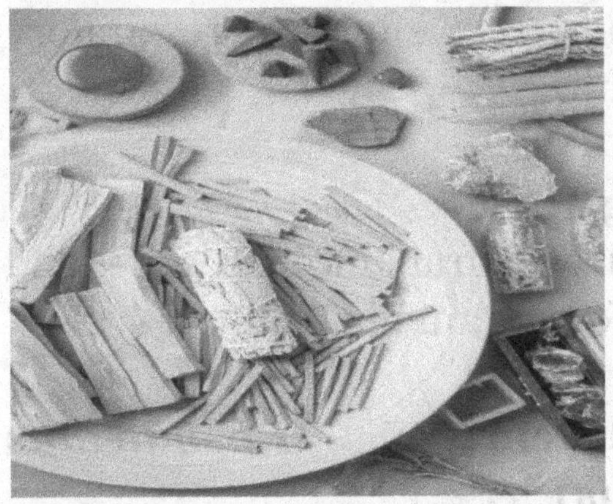

Botanical Name: *Santalum album*

Main Properties:
- **Grounding**: Promotes relaxation and meditation.
- **Anti-inflammatory**: Soothes irritated skin.

- **Antiseptic**: Cleanses and heals minor wounds.

Uses and Benefits:

- **Meditation Aid:** Diffuse during meditation or prayer for grounding.
- **Skin Health:** Apply diluted oil to soothe and heal skin.
- **Respiratory Support**: Use in blends to support respiratory health.

Blending Tips:
Pairs well with frankincense, rose, and lavender for a calming blend.

14. Rosemary (*Rosmarinus officinalis*)

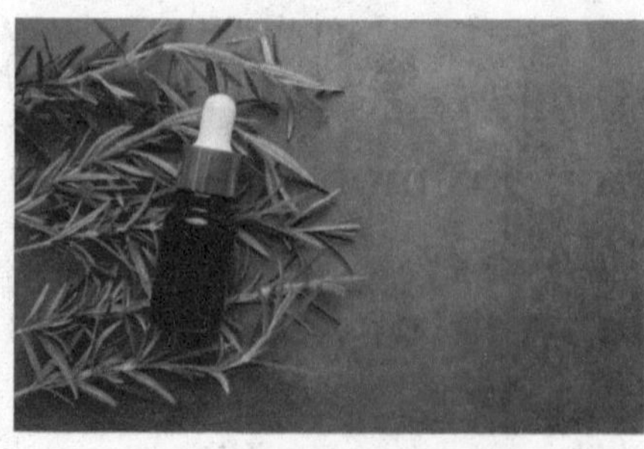

Botanical Name: *Rosmarinus officinalis*

Main Properties:
- **Stimulating**: Enhances memory and focus.
- **Antimicrobial**: Fights bacterial infections.
- **Antioxidant**: Protects against free radical damage.

Uses and Benefits:
- **Mental Clarity**: Diffuse to enhance focus and memory.
- **Hair Health**: Apply diluted oil to the scalp to promote hair growth.
- **Respiratory Support**: Use in blends for respiratory health.

Blending Tips:
Mix with peppermint, eucalyptus, and lemon for an invigorating blend.

15. Jasmine (*Jasminum officinale*)

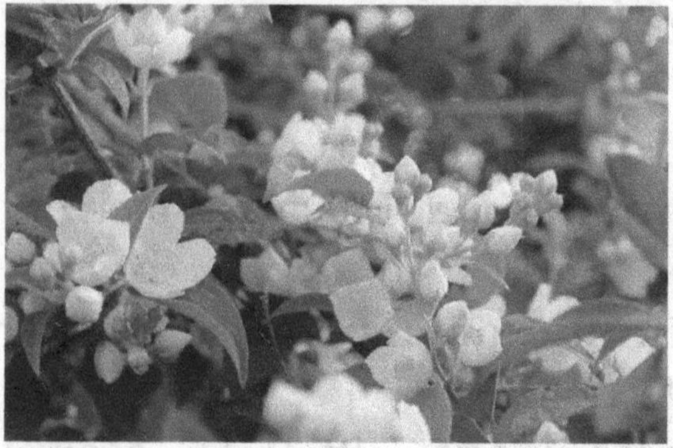

Botanical Name: *Jasminum officinale*

Main Properties:

- **Antidepressant**: Uplifts mood and soothes emotions.
- **Antispasmodic**: Eases muscle spasms and cramps.
- **Aphrodisiac**: Enhances romantic moods.

Uses and Benefits:

- **Emotional Well-being**: Diffuse to uplift and soothe emotions.
- **Skin Care:** Use in blends to improve skin tone and texture.
- **Aphrodisiac**: Diffuse to enhance romantic moods.

Blending Tips:
Blends well with ylang-ylang, sandalwood, and citrus oils for a luxurious scent.

16. Patchouli (*Pogostemon cablin*)

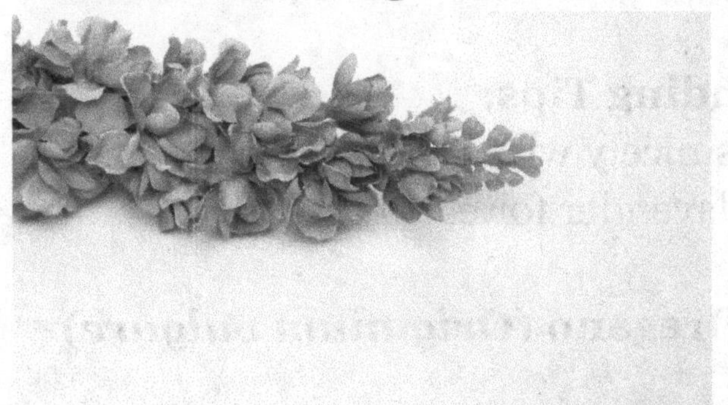

Botanical Name: *Pogostemon cablin*

Main Properties:
- **Grounding**: Promotes relaxation and reduces stress.
- **Anti-inflammatory**: Reduces skin inflammation.
- **Antiseptic**: Cleanses and heals minor wounds.

Uses and Benefits:

- **Stress Relief**: Diffuse or apply diluted oil to reduce anxiety.
- **Skin Care**: Use in blends to soothe and heal skin.
- **Insect Repellent**: Add to homemade insect repellents.

Blending Tips:

Pairs nicely with sandalwood, bergamot, and lavender for earthy blends.

17. Oregano (*Origanum vulgare*)

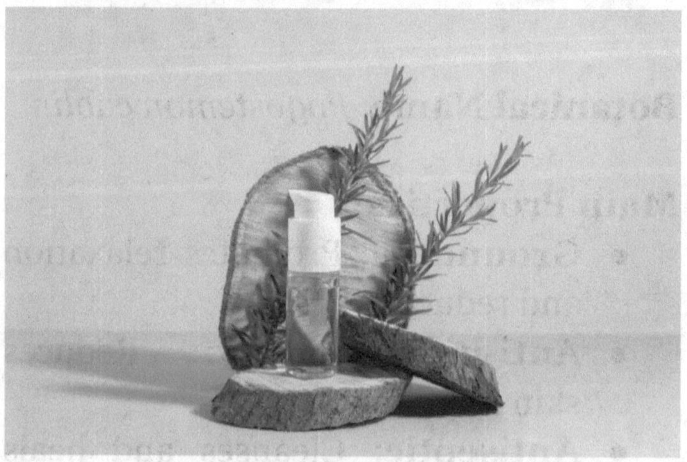

Botanical Name: *Origanum vulgare*

Main Properties:

- **Antimicrobial**: Fights bacterial, viral, and fungal infections.
- **Anti-inflammatory**: Reduces inflammation.
- **Immune-boosting**: Supports immune health.

Uses and Benefits:

- **Infection Fighter**: Use in blends to fight infections.
- **Immune Support**: Diffuse or apply diluted oil to boost immune function.
- **Muscle Pain Relief**: Apply diluted oil to sore muscles to reduce pain and inflammation.

Blending Tips:

Use sparingly and blend with tea tree, eucalyptus, and rosemary for powerful antimicrobial effects.

18. Cypress (*Cupressus sempervirens*)

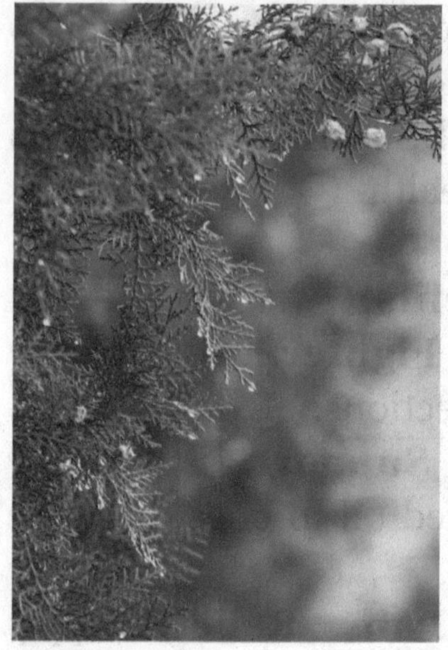

Botanical Name: *Cupressus sempervirens*

Main Properties:
- **Astringent**: Tightens and tones skin.
- **Antiseptic**: Cleanses and heals minor wounds.
- **Antispasmodic**: Eases muscle spasms and cramps.

Uses and Benefits:

- **Respiratory Health**: Diffuse to support breathing and ease respiratory issues.
- **Pain Relief**: Apply diluted oil to areas of swelling and pain to reduce discomfort.
- **Circulation**: Use in blends to promote healthy circulation.

Blending Tips:
Blends well with lavender, bergamot, and juniper for respiratory support and skin care.

19. Grapefruit (*Citrus paradisi*)

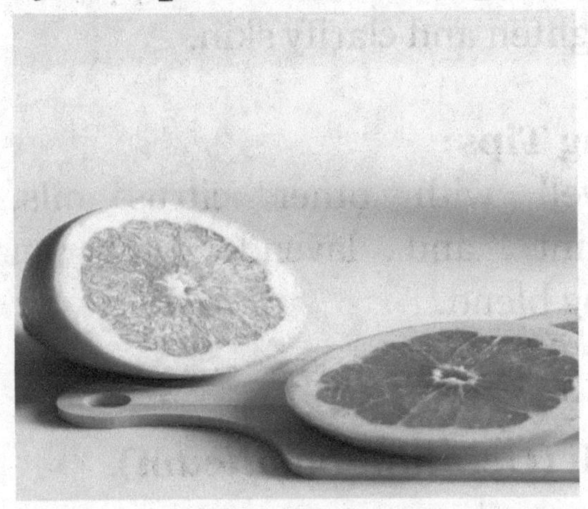

Botanical Name: *Citrus paradisi*

Main Properties:
- **Uplifting**: Enhances mood and energy.
- **Antiseptic**: Cleanses and purifies.
- **Detoxifying**: Supports the body's detox processes.

Uses and Benefits:
- **Mood Booster**: Diffuse to uplift and energize.
- **Cleaning**: Add to homemade cleaning products for its antibacterial properties.
- **Skin Care**: Dilute and apply to brighten and clarify skin.

Blending Tips:
Pairs well with other citrus oils, peppermint, and lavender for an energizing blend.

20. Basil (*Ocimum basilicum*)

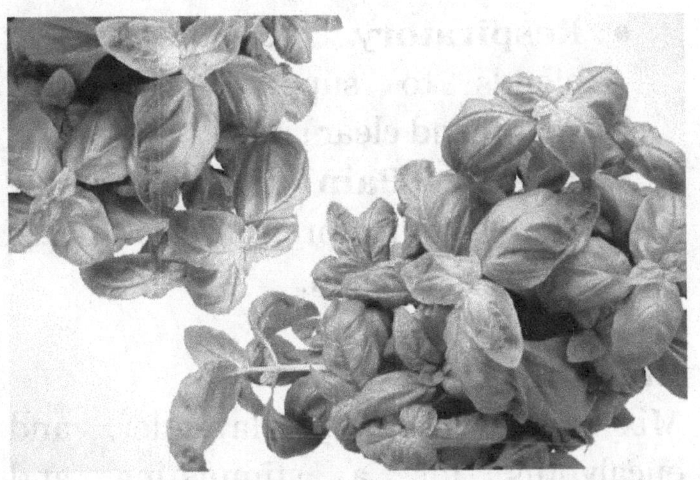

Botanical Name: *Ocimum basilicum*

Main Properties:

- **Stimulating**: Enhances mental clarity and focus.
- **Antimicrobial**: Fights bacterial infections.
- **Antispasmodic**: Eases muscle spasms and cramps.

Uses and Benefits:

- **Mental Clarity:** Diffuse to enhance focus and concentration.

- **Respiratory Health**: Use in blends to support respiratory health and clear sinuses.
- **Muscle Pain Relief**: Apply diluted oil to sore muscles to ease spasms and pain.

Blending Tips:
Mix with rosemary, lavender, and eucalyptus for a stimulating and clarifying blend.

These 20 essential oils provide a broad spectrum of benefits and uses for beginners. By understanding each oil's properties and how to use them effectively, you can add essential oils into your daily routine for improved physical health, emotional well-being, and overall quality of life. Remember to always follow safety guidelines, including proper dilution and patch testing, to ensure you use essential oils safely and effectively.

Chapter 4:

Methods of Use

Essential oils can be enjoyed in many different ways, each offering unique benefits. Understanding these methods will help you make the most of your essential oils. In this chapter, we'll explore various ways to use essential oils, including aromatherapy, diffusers, inhalation techniques, and aromatherapy jewelry.

Aromatherapy

Aromatherapy is the practice of using essential oils to enhance physical and emotional well-being. The oils are either inhaled or applied to the skin. Here's how aromatherapy works and how you can use it effectively:

Inhalation: Breathing in the aroma of essential oils can have immediate effects on the brain, particularly the limbic system, which controls emotions and memories. This can help with stress relief, mood enhancement, and even physical benefits like improved respiratory function.

Topical Application: Applying diluted essential oils to the skin allows them to be absorbed into the bloodstream. This can be beneficial for localized pain relief, skin care, and overall relaxation.

Diffusers and Humidifiers

Using a diffuser is one of the most popular methods for enjoying essential oils. There are several types of diffusers, each with its advantages:

1. **Ultrasonic Diffusers**: These use water and ultrasonic waves to disperse essential oils into the air as a fine mist.

They also act as humidifiers, adding moisture to the air, which can be especially beneficial in dry climates.

2. Nebulizing Diffusers: These do not use water or heat. Instead, they use an atomizer to create fine particles of essential oil, offering a powerful and pure diffusion. They are great for large areas and for getting the maximum therapeutic benefits from your oils.

3. Evaporative Diffusers: These use a fan to blow air through a pad or filter that has been saturated with essential oil. As the oil evaporates, its aroma is dispersed into the air. They are typically less expensive but may not be as effective for therapeutic use.

4. Heat Diffusers: These use heat, such as a candle or an electric heating element, to gently evaporate the essential oils into the air. They are simple and quiet but can alter the chemical composition of the oils due to the heat.

How to Use Diffusers:
- Fill the diffuser with water (if required) up to the indicated level.
- Add 5-10 drops of your chosen essential oil.
- Turn on the diffuser and enjoy the aromatic benefits.

Inhalation Techniques

Inhalation is a straightforward and effective way to experience the benefits of essential oils. Here are some common techniques:

1. Direct Inhalation: Simply open a bottle of essential oil and take a few deep breaths. This method is quick and effective for immediate results, such as reducing stress or clearing sinuses.

2. Steam Inhalation: Add a few drops of essential oil to a bowl of hot water, place a towel over your head, and inhale the steam. This method is particularly beneficial for respiratory issues and deep relaxation.

3. Tissue or Cotton Ball: Put a few drops of essential oil on a tissue or cotton ball and place it near your nose. This is a convenient method for when you're on the go.

Safety Tip: Always keep your eyes closed during steam inhalation to avoid irritation.

Aromatherapy Jewelry

Aromatherapy jewelry is a fashionable and portable way to enjoy the benefits of essential oils throughout the day. Here's how it works and how you can use it:

1. **Diffuser Necklaces**: These necklaces typically have a locket or a small chamber that holds a felt pad, lava stone, or another absorbent material. You add a few drops of essential oil to the material, which slowly releases the aroma.

2. Diffuser Bracelets: Similar to necklaces, these bracelets often use absorbent beads or pads that can be infused with essential oils. Wearing them on your wrist allows you to enjoy the benefits throughout the day.

3. Diffuser Earrings: Some earrings are designed with small absorbent beads or pads that can hold essential oils. They provide a subtle way to enjoy aromatherapy.

How to Use Aromatherapy Jewelry:

- Apply 1-2 drops of essential oil to the absorbent material.

- Allow the oil to absorb and dry slightly before wearing the jewelry.
- Reapply as needed throughout the day.

Benefits of Aromatherapy Jewelry:
- Portable and convenient, allowing you to enjoy essential oils on the go.
- Fashionable and discreet, making it easy to incorporate into your daily routine.
- Personal and customizable, letting you choose the oils that suit your needs.

There are many ways to incorporate essential oils into your daily life, from using diffusers and humidifiers to practicing inhalation techniques and wearing aromatherapy jewelry. Each method has its unique benefits and can be chosen based on your personal preferences and needs. Whether you're looking to create a relaxing home environment, alleviate stress, or boost your mood, there's a method of use that's perfect for you. Remember to always use essential oils safely and follow guidelines for dilution and application to maximize their benefits.

Topical Application

Applying essential oils directly to the skin is known as topical application. This method allows the oils to be absorbed into the bloodstream and can target specific areas of the body. When using essential oils topically, it's important to dilute them properly to avoid skin irritation. Here's an extensive look into how to use essential oils topically through massage oils and lotions, compresses and poultices, and skincare and beauty routines.

Massage Oils and Lotions

Massage Oils: One of the most common ways to use essential oils topically is through massage oils. Massage combines the therapeutic benefits of essential oils with the relaxing effects of physical touch.

Making Massage Oil:
- Choose a carrier oil such as coconut, jojoba, almond, or olive oil.
- Add 10-15 drops of essential oil per ounce of carrier oil. Some good options include lavender for relaxation, peppermint for muscle pain, or eucalyptus for respiratory benefits.
- Mix well and store in a dark glass bottle.

How to Use:
- Warm the oil by rubbing it between your hands.

- Apply the oil to the skin and use gentle, circular motions to massage the area.
- Focus on areas of tension, such as the neck, shoulders, back, and feet.

Lotions: Adding essential oils to lotions can enhance their moisturizing and therapeutic properties.

Making Aromatherapy Lotion:
- Choose a natural, unscented lotion.
- Add 10-15 drops of essential oil per ounce of lotion. Consider using chamomile for soothing irritated skin, tea tree for its antiseptic properties, or geranium for balancing the skin.
- Mix thoroughly and store in a clean container.

<u>How to Use:</u>

- Apply the lotion as you would normally, focusing on dry or irritated areas.
- Use daily for best results.

Compresses and Poultices

Compresses and poultices are effective for treating localized pain, inflammation, and infections.

Compresses: A compress is a cloth soaked in water and essential oils that is applied to the skin.

Making a Compress:
- Fill a bowl with warm or cold water, depending on the treatment needed (warm for muscle relaxation, cold for inflammation).
- Add 5-10 drops of essential oil to the water. For example, lavender and chamomile are great for relaxation, while peppermint and

eucalyptus can help with pain and inflammation.

- Soak a clean cloth in the mixture, wring out the excess water, and apply the cloth to the affected area.

How to Use:

- Leave the compress on the area for about 15-20 minutes.
- Repeat as needed, using fresh water and oils each time.

Poultices: A poultice is a paste made from herbs and essential oils, applied to the skin, and covered with a cloth.

Making a Poultice:

- Mix powdered herbs (such as chamomile, comfrey, or turmeric) with a few drops of essential oil and enough water to make a thick paste.
- Apply the paste to the affected area.

- Cover with a clean cloth or bandage to keep the poultice in place.

How to Use:
- Leave the poultice on for about 20-30 minutes.
- Remove and rinse the area with warm water.
- Repeat as needed for best results.

Skincare and Beauty

Essential oils can be a wonderful addition to your skincare and beauty routine, offering a natural way to care for your skin.

Facial Serums and Oils:

Making Facial Serum:
- Choose a carrier oil suitable for your skin type, such as argan oil

for dry skin or jojoba oil for oily skin.

- Add 5-10 drops of essential oil per ounce of carrier oil. Consider using frankincense for anti-aging, tea tree for acne, or rose for moisturizing.
- Mix well and store in a dropper bottle.

How to Use:
- Apply a few drops to your face after cleansing and before moisturizing.
- Gently massage into the skin using upward, circular motions.

Toners:

Making Toner:
- Mix 1 part witch hazel with 1 part distilled water.
- Add 5-10 drops of essential oil per ounce of liquid. Lavender and chamomile are excellent for

soothing the skin, while tea tree is good for acne-prone skin.

- Store in a spray bottle or an airtight container.

How to Use:

- After cleansing, apply the toner to a cotton pad and swipe over your face, or spritz directly onto the skin.
- Follow with your regular skincare routine.

Body Scrubs:

Making Body Scrub:

- Combine 1 cup of sugar or salt with 1/2 cup of a carrier oil.
- Add 10-15 drops of essential oil. For example, grapefruit and rosemary are invigorating, while lavender and chamomile are calming.
- Mix well and store in a jar.

<u>**How to Use:**</u>
- In the shower, apply the scrub to damp skin.
- Gently massage in circular motions, focusing on rough areas like elbows, knees, and feet.
- Rinse thoroughly and pat dry.

Hair Care:

Hair Oil:
- Mix a carrier oil (such as coconut or argan oil) with 5-10 drops of essential oil per ounce of carrier oil. Rosemary and peppermint are great for hair growth, while lavender and chamomile can soothe the scalp.
- Store in a dark glass bottle.

<u>**How to Use:**</u>
- Apply a small amount to your scalp and hair, focusing on the ends.

- Leave in for at least 30 minutes or overnight, then wash out with shampoo.

Hair Rinse:
- Add a few drops of essential oil to a cup of water or apple cider vinegar.
- Use as a final rinse after shampooing and conditioning.

Internal Use

Using essential oils internally can offer various benefits, but it's essential to approach this method with caution and proper knowledge. In this section, we'll cover how to use essential oils in cooking, as supplements and capsules, and the important safety considerations to keep in mind.

Cooking with Essential Oils

Adding essential oils to your cooking can be a great way to enhance flavors and enjoy their health benefits. However, because essential oils are highly concentrated, a little goes a long way.

How to Cook with Essential Oils:

1. Start Small: Use only a drop or two. Essential oils are much stronger than dried or fresh herbs and spices.

2. Mix with Fat: Dilute the essential oil in a cooking oil, butter, or another fat source before adding it to your dish. This helps distribute the oil evenly and enhances its flavor.

3. Add at the End: To preserve the beneficial properties of essential oils, add them towards the end of cooking, especially if they are heat-sensitive.

Examples of Essential Oils that can be used in Cooking:

- **Peppermint oil**: Great for desserts like brownies, cakes, and hot chocolate.
- Lemon oil: Adds a fresh, zesty flavor to salad dressings, marinades, and baked goods.
- Basil oil: Enhances pasta sauces, soups, and salads.
- **Oregano**: Perfect for Italian dishes like pizza and pasta sauces.

<u>Safety Tip</u>: Not all essential oils are safe for consumption. Ensure you use only food-grade essential oils and verify their safety for internal use.

Supplements and Capsules

Essential oils can also be taken internally in the form of supplements and capsules. This method can target specific health issues and provide concentrated benefits. However, it's crucial to do this correctly to avoid potential side effects.

How to Use Essential Oil Supplements:

1. Consult a Professional: Always talk to a healthcare provider or a certified aromatherapist before taking essential oils internally. They can help you determine the right dosage and oil for your needs.
2. Use Quality Products: Only use essential oils that are labeled as safe for internal use and are of high quality and purity.
3. Follow Dosage Instructions: Stick to the recommended dosage. Taking too much can lead to toxicity and adverse reactions.

Making Essential Oil Capsules:

1. Choose Your Oil: Select an essential oil that is safe for internal use, such as peppermint for digestive support or frankincense for immune support.

2. Dilute Properly: Mix the essential oil with a carrier oil, such as olive oil, in a safe ratio (typically 1-2 drops of essential oil per capsule).

3. Fill Capsules: Use empty gel capsules, available at health food stores, and fill them with the diluted essential oil mixture.

4. Take with Food: To avoid stomach irritation, take the capsule with food.

Safety Considerations

Using essential oils internally requires strict adherence to safety guidelines to prevent adverse effects. Here are some key points to keep in mind:

1. **Quality Matters:** Ensure you use high-quality, therapeutic-grade essential oils that are safe for internal use. Poor-quality oils may contain harmful additives or contaminants.

2. Know the Oils: Not all essential oils are safe for ingestion. Oils like eucalyptus, wintergreen, and tea tree should never be taken internally due to their potential toxicity.

3. Dilution is Crucial: Always dilute essential oils before consuming. Taking undiluted oils can cause serious health issues, including burns, irritation, and toxicity.

4. Be Aware of Interactions: Essential oils can interact with medications and medical conditions. Always consult with a healthcare provider if you're taking medications or have any health concerns.

5. Monitor for Reactions: Be vigilant about any adverse reactions, such as digestive discomfort, headaches, or allergic reactions. If you experience any negative symptoms, stop using the essential oil immediately and seek medical advice.

Chapter 5:

Creating Your Own Blends

Creating your own essential oil blends can be a rewarding and creative process. Blending allows you to tailor the therapeutic properties and aromas to your personal needs and preferences. In this chapter, we'll cover the basics of blending, understanding the different notes in essential oils, the concept of synergy and balance, and how to measure and record your blends.

Basics of Blending

Blending essential oils involves mixing different oils to create a harmonious and effective combination. Here are some basic guidelines to get you started:

1. Start Simple: Begin with just a few oils—two or three—until you become more comfortable with the process.

2. Know Your Oils: Familiarize yourself with the properties and scents of individual oils. This helps you understand how they might work together.

3. Dilution: Always dilute your blends with a carrier oil, especially if you plan to use them topically. A common dilution ratio is 1-2% for adults, which means about 5-10 drops of essential oil per ounce of carrier oil.

Understanding Notes: (Top, Middle, and Base):

Essential oils can be categorized into three main notes: top, middle, and base. Each note plays a role in the blend's aroma and therapeutic effects.

Top Notes:

Characteristics: Light, fresh, and uplifting.

Evaporation Rate: Fast (they evaporate quickly).

Examples: Lemon, peppermint, eucalyptus.

Role in Blends: These oils are often the first scent you notice and they tend to evaporate quickly. They provide an initial impression and can lift your mood.

Middle Notes:

Characteristics: Warm, soft, and balancing.

Evaporation Rate: Moderate.

Examples: Lavender, chamomile, rosemary.

Role in Blends: Middle notes create the heart of the blend. They add balance and complexity, often providing the therapeutic benefits.

Base Notes:

Characteristics: Deep, rich, and grounding.

Evaporation Rate: Slow (they linger the longest).

Examples: Frankincense, sandalwood, patchouli.

Role in Blends: Base notes add depth and longevity to a blend. They ground and anchor the scent, making it last longer.

When blending, aim for a balanced mix of these notes. A typical blend might include 30% top notes, 50% middle notes, and 20% base notes, but you can adjust this based on your preference and the intended use of the blend.

Synergy and Balance

Synergy is the idea that the combined effect of the oils in a blend is greater than the sum of their individual effects. A well-balanced blend can enhance the therapeutic properties of each oil.

Creating Synergy

Choose Complementary Oils: Select oils that work well together both therapeutically and aromatically. For example, lavender and chamomile both have calming properties and blend well together.

Experiment: Try different combinations and ratios to find what works best for you. Sometimes unexpected pairings can create the most delightful and effective blends.

Achieving Balance

Consider the Purpose: Think about what you want the blend to achieve. Are you looking for relaxation, energy, or a specific health benefit?

Adjust Ratios: Start with small amounts and adjust the ratios until you find the perfect balance. A balanced blend should smell harmonious and provide the desired effect without any one oil overpowering the others.

Measuring and Recording Blends

Keeping track of your blends is crucial, especially when you create something you love and want to replicate it in the future.

Measuring:
- **Use Droppers**: Essential oils are typically measured in drops. Use a dropper to ensure precision.
- **Create Small Batches**: Start with small amounts (e.g., a 10 ml bottle) so you can experiment without wasting oils.
- **Convert Measurements**: If you need larger quantities, convert the drop measurements to milliliters or ounces accurately.

Recording:

- **Label Your Blends:** Always label your bottles with the name of the blend, the date, and the ingredients with their proportions.

- **Keep a Journal**: Write down each blend you create, noting the oils used, their ratios, and your impressions. Include how the blend smells initially and over time, as well as its effects.

- **Review and Refine**: Use your notes to refine your blends. Adjust the proportions if needed and document any changes for future reference.

Creating your own essential oil blends is a blend of art and science. By understanding the basics of blending, the different notes, and the principles of synergy and balance, you can craft personalized and effective essential oil blends. Always measure carefully and keep detailed records of your creations to ensure you can replicate or adjust them as needed. With practice and experimentation, you'll develop a deeper understanding of how to create harmonious and beneficial blends tailored to your needs.

Blending for Specific Purposes

Creating essential oil blends tailored for specific purposes can enhance their effectiveness and provide targeted benefits. In this section, we'll explore how to blend essential oils for relaxation and stress relief, energy and focus, sleep and insomnia, pain and inflammation, skin care and beauty, and cleaning and disinfecting.

Relaxation and Stress Relief

Essential oils can be incredibly effective for promoting relaxation and reducing stress. Here are some oils and blends that are particularly good for this purpose:

1. **Lavender oil**: Known for its calming and soothing properties.
2. **Chamomile oil**: Offers a gentle, relaxing effect.
3. **Bergamot oil**: Helps to uplift mood while calming the mind.
4. **Frankincense oil**: Promotes deep relaxation and mental clarity.

Relaxation Blend:
- 5 drops Lavender oil
- 3 drops Chamomile oil
- 2 drops Bergamot oil
- 1 drop Frankincense oil

How to Use:
Diffuser: Add 5-10 drops of the blend to your diffuser.

Massage Oil: Dilute 10 drops of the blend in 1 ounce of carrier oil.

Bath: Add 5-10 drops of the blend to a warm bath.

Energy and Focus

When you need a boost of energy or improved concentration, essential oils can help invigorate your senses and sharpen your mind. Examples includes:

- **Peppermint oil**: Stimulates the mind and boosts energy.
- Rosemary oil: Enhances memory and cognitive function.
- **Lemon oil**: Provides a refreshing and uplifting effect.
- **Eucalyptus oil**: Helps clear the mind and improve focus.

Energy and Focus Blend:
- 5 drops Peppermint oil
- 4 drops Rosemary oil

- 3 drops Lemon oil
- 2 drops Eucalyptus oil

How to Use:
- **Diffuser**: Add 5-10 drops of the blend to your diffuser.
- **Inhalation**: Put a few drops on a tissue or cotton ball and inhale deeply.
- **Roller Bottle**: Combine 10 drops of the blend with 1 ounce of carrier oil in a roller bottle for easy application on the go.

Sleep and Insomnia

For those struggling with sleep issues, certain essential oils can help you unwind and prepare for a restful night. Examples are:
- **Lavender oil**: Promotes relaxation and improves sleep quality.

- Cedarwood oil: Has a calming and grounding effect.
- **Roman Chamomile oil**: Helps soothe the mind and body.
- **Marjoram oil**: Encourages relaxation and sleep.

Sleep Blend:
- 6 drops Lavender
- 4 drops Cedarwood
- 3 drops Roman Chamomile
- 2 drops Marjoram

How to Use:
- **Diffuser**: Add 5-10 drops of the blend to your diffuser an hour before bedtime.
- **Pillow Spray**: Mix 10 drops of the blend with 2 ounces of water in a spray bottle and spritz your pillow.
- **Massage Oil**: Dilute 10 drops of the blend in 1 ounce of carrier oil and massage into your feet or shoulders.

Pain and Inflammation

Essential oils can be powerful allies in managing pain and reducing inflammation. Such oil includes:

- **Peppermint oil**: Provides a cooling sensation and relieves pain.
- **Eucalyptus oil**: Reduces inflammation and soothes aches.
- **Lavender oil**: Offers calming and anti-inflammatory properties.
- **Ginger oil**: Warms and soothes sore muscles.

Pain and Inflammation Blend:
- 5 drops Peppermint oil
- 4 drops Eucalyptus oil
- 3 drops Lavender oil
- 2 drops Ginger oil

How to Use:
- **Massage Oil:** Dilute 10 drops of the blend in 1 ounce of carrier oil and massage into affected areas.

- **Compress**: Add 5-10 drops of the blend to a bowl of warm water, soak a cloth, and apply to the painful area.
- **Bath**: Add 5-10 drops of the blend to a warm bath.

Skin Care and Beauty

Essential oils can enhance your skincare routine, providing natural solutions for various skin concerns. Examples are:
- **Tea Tree oil:** Antiseptic and great for acne-prone skin.
- **Frankincense oil:** Promotes cell regeneration and reduces scars.
- **Geranium oil**: Balances oil production and improves complexion.
- **Lavender oil**: Soothes and heals the skin.

Skincare Blend:
- 5 drops Tea Tree oil

- 4 drops Frankincense oil
- 3 drops Geranium oil
- 2 drops Lavender oil

How to Use:
- **Facial Serum:** Dilute 10 drops of the blend in 1 ounce of carrier oil like jojoba or argan oil. Apply a few drops to your face after cleansing.
- **Face Mask:** Add a few drops of the blend to your favorite clay or honey mask.
- **Spot Treatment:** Dilute 1-2 drops of the blend in a teaspoon of carrier oil and apply to blemishes.

Cleaning and Disinfecting

Essential oils can be effective natural cleaners due to their antimicrobial properties. Some examples include:

- **Lemon oil**: Antibacterial and cuts through grease.
- **Tea Tree oil**: Antiseptic and disinfectant.
- **Eucalyptus oil:** Antimicrobial and fresh-smelling.
- **Peppermint oil**: Antibacterial and leaves a fresh scent.

Cleaning Blend:
- 5 drops Lemon oil
- 4 drops Tea Tree oil
- 3 drops Eucalyptus oil
- 2 drops Peppermint oil

How to Use:
- All-Purpose Cleaner: Mix 10-15 drops of the blend with 1 cup of water and 1 cup of white vinegar in a spray bottle. Shake well before each use.
- **Surface Spray**: Combine 10 drops of the blend with 2 cups of water in a spray bottle for a natural disinfectant.

- **Floor Cleaner**: Add 10 drops of the blend to a bucket of warm water and use it to mop floors.

Blending essential oils for specific purposes allows you to create customized solutions for a variety of needs, from relaxation and sleep to energy and cleaning. By understanding the properties of different oils and how to combine them effectively, you can maximize their benefits and enhance your well-being. Always remember to use essential oils safely, diluting them properly and testing blends before extensive use.

Chapter 6:

Essential Oils for Health and Wellness

Essential oils offer a natural and holistic approach to supporting health and wellness. They can be used to address common ailments, boost the immune system, and support respiratory health. Let's explore various physical health applications of essential oils, focusing on their use for headaches, colds, muscle pain, immune support, and respiratory health.

Physical Health Applications

Essential oils can be highly effective in managing a variety of physical health issues. Here, we'll cover some of the most common ailments and how essential oils can help.

Common Ailments:

1. Headaches:

Peppermint Oil: Known for its cooling effect, peppermint oil can help alleviate tension headaches. Apply diluted peppermint oil to the temples and back of the neck for relief.

Lavender Oil: This oil is excellent for stress-related headaches due to its calming properties. Diffuse lavender oil or apply it topically to the temples.

Eucalyptus Oil: Useful for sinus headaches, eucalyptus oil can help clear nasal passages. Inhale it through steam or apply diluted to the chest and temples.

Headache Relief Blend:
- 3 drops Peppermint Oil
- 3 drops Lavender Oil
- 2 drops Eucalyptus Oil

<u>**How to Use:**</u>

- **Topical Application**: Dilute the blend with a carrier oil (such as coconut or jojoba oil) and apply to the temples, neck, and shoulders.
- **Inhalation**: Add a few drops to a bowl of hot water, cover your head with a towel, and inhale the steam.

2. Colds:

Eucalyptus Oil: Its antiviral and decongestant properties make it great for relieving cold symptoms. Diffuse eucalyptus oil or add it to a steam inhalation.

Tea Tree Oil: With its antimicrobial properties, tea tree oil can help fight off infections. Add a few drops to a bowl of hot water for steam inhalation.

Peppermint Oil: Helps to clear nasal passages and reduce congestion. Apply diluted peppermint oil to the chest or inhale it directly.

Cold Relief Blend:
- 4 drops Eucalyptus Oil

- 3 drops Tea Tree Oil
- 3 drops Peppermint Oil

How to Use:

- **Steam Inhalation**: Add a few drops of the blend to a bowl of hot water, cover your head with a towel, and inhale deeply.
- **Chest Rub**: Dilute the blend with a carrier oil and apply to the chest and throat.

3. Muscle Pain:

Peppermint Oil:Its cooling and anti-inflammatory properties can help relieve muscle pain. Apply diluted peppermint oil to sore muscles.

Lavender Oil: Offers calming and anti-inflammatory benefits, making it great for muscle relaxation. Use it in a massage oil blend.

Eucalyptus Oil: Helps reduce inflammation and soothe sore muscles. Apply diluted oil to the affected area.

Muscle Pain Relief Blend:
- 4 drops Peppermint Oil
- 4 drops Lavender Oil
- 2 drops Eucalyptus Oil

How to Use:
- **Massage Oil**: Dilute the blend with a carrier oil and massage into sore muscles.
- **Bath Soak**: Add a few drops of the blend to a warm bath for overall muscle relaxation.

Immune System Support

Essential oils can play a significant role in supporting and boosting the immune system. Their antimicrobial, antiviral, and anti-inflammatory properties help protect the body from illnesses.

Immune-Boosting Oils:
Tea Tree Oil: Known for its powerful antimicrobial properties, tea tree oil can help fight off infections.

Eucalyptus Oil: Supports respiratory health and has antiviral properties.
Frankincense Oil: Boosts the immune system and reduces inflammation.
Lemon Oil: Its high vitamin C content and antioxidant properties support immune health.

Immune Support Blend:
- 4 drops Tea Tree Oil
- 4 drops Eucalyptus Oil
- 3 drops Frankincense Oil
- 3 drops Lemon Oil

<u>How to Use:</u>
- **Diffusion**: Add 5-10 drops of the blend to a diffuser to purify the air and support immune health.
- **Topical Application**: Dilute the blend with a carrier oil and apply to the soles of the feet, back of the neck, and chest.

Respiratory Health

Essential oils can be particularly beneficial for maintaining and improving respiratory health. They help clear airways, reduce inflammation, and combat infections.

Respiratory Health Oils:

Eucalyptus Oil: Known for its ability to open airways and reduce inflammation, making it ideal for respiratory issues.

Peppermint Oil:Helps clear nasal passages and reduce congestion.

Tea Tree Oil: Offers antimicrobial properties that can help fight respiratory infections.

Lavender Oil: Soothes the respiratory system and can be used to relieve symptoms of asthma and bronchitis.

Respiratory Support Blend:
- 5 drops Eucalyptus Oil
- 4 drops Peppermint Oil

- 3 drops Tea Tree Oil
- 3 drops Lavender Oil

How to Use:

- **Steam Inhalation**: Add a few drops of the blend to a bowl of hot water, cover your head with a towel, and inhale deeply to clear nasal passages and soothe the respiratory system.
- **Chest Rub**: Dilute the blend with a carrier oil and apply to the chest and throat to help with congestion and breathing.

Mental and Emotional Wellness

Essential oils can have a profound impact on mental and emotional wellness. They offer natural support for relieving stress and anxiety, enhancing mood, and improving cognitive function and concentration. In this section, we will explore how specific essential oils can be used to address these areas and provide practical ways to incorporate them into your daily routine.

Stress and Anxiety Relief

In our fast-paced world, stress and anxiety are common issues that many people face. Essential oils can provide a natural and effective way to manage these feelings and promote relaxation.

Key Oils for Stress and Anxiety Relief:

Lavender oil: Known for its calming and soothing properties, lavender is one of the most popular oils for reducing stress and anxiety.

Bergamot oil: This citrus oil has mood-lifting and calming effects, helping to alleviate anxiety and stress.

Chamomile Oi: Offers a gentle, calming effect that can help reduce stress and promote relaxation.

Frankincense oil: Known for its grounding properties, frankincense can help calm the mind and reduce feelings of anxiety.

Stress and Anxiety Relief Blend:
- 5 drops Lavender oil
- 4 drops Bergamot oil
- 3 drops Chamomile oil
- 2 drops Frankincense oil

How to Use:
- **Diffuser**: Add 5-10 drops of the blend to your diffuser. This can help create a calming atmosphere in your home or workspace.
- **Topical Application**: Dilute the blend with a carrier oil (such as coconut or almond oil) and apply it to your wrists, temples, and the back of your neck.
- **Inhalation**: Put a few drops on a cotton ball or tissue and inhale deeply whenever you feel stressed or anxious.

Mood Enhancement

Essential oils can be powerful tools for lifting your mood and promoting feelings of happiness and well-being. Whether you're feeling down or simply want to maintain a positive outlook, these oils can help.

Key Oils for Mood Enhancement:
Lemon oil: This bright and cheerful oil is known for its ability to uplift the mood and energize the spirit.
Orange oil: Another citrus favorite, orange oil has a sweet, refreshing scent that can help dispel feelings of sadness and promote a positive mood.
Ylang-Ylang oil: This floral oil has balancing properties that can help uplift the mood and reduce feelings of sadness.
Rose oil: Known for its luxurious and uplifting aroma, rose oil can help improve mood and alleviate feelings of depression.

Mood Enhancement Blend:

- 5 drops Lemon oil
- 4 drops Orange oil
- 3 drops Ylang-Ylang oil
- 2 drops Rose oil

How to Use:

- **Diffuser**: Add 5-10 drops of the blend to your diffuser to fill your space with a cheerful, uplifting aroma.
- **Inhalation**: Carry a personal inhaler or a small bottle of the blend with you to use throughout the day.
- **Bath**: Add a few drops of the blend to a warm bath for a relaxing and mood-enhancing soak.

Cognitive Function and Concentration

Maintaining focus and enhancing cognitive function is crucial, whether you're studying, working, or simply trying to stay sharp. Essential oils can provide a natural boost to your mental clarity and concentration.

Key Oils for Cognitive Function and Concentration:

Peppermint oil: This invigorating oil helps stimulate the mind and improve focus and concentration.

Rosemary oil: Known for its memory-enhancing properties, rosemary oil can help improve cognitive function and mental clarity.

Lemon: Helps to clear the mind and improve concentration, making it easier to focus on tasks.

Basil: This herbaceous oil is great for enhancing mental alertness and reducing mental fatigue.

Cognitive Function and Concentration Blend:
- 5 drops Peppermint oil

- 4 drops Rosemary oil
- 3 drops Lemon oil
- 2 drops Basil oil

How to Use:

- **Diffuser**: Add 5-10 drops of the blend to your diffuser to create an environment conducive to focus and productivity.

- **Topical Application**: Dilute the blend with a carrier oil and apply it to your temples, back of the neck, and wrists before starting a task that requires concentration.

- **Inhalation**: Use a personal inhaler or put a few drops on a tissue and inhale deeply to help maintain focus throughout the day.

Practical Tips for Using Essential Oils for Mental and Emotional Wellness

1. **Create a Routine**: Incorporate essential oils into your daily routine to

maximize their benefits. For example, use calming oils in the evening to unwind or energizing oils in the morning to start your day with focus.

2. Personalize Your Blends: Experiment with different oils and ratios to find what works best for you. Everyone's response to essential oils is unique, so personalizing your blends can enhance their effectiveness.

3. Use Safe Practices: Always dilute essential oils before applying them to the skin and perform a patch test to check for any adverse reactions. Avoid using oils that you are allergic to or that may interact with any medications you are taking.

4. Stay Consistent: Consistency is key to experiencing the full benefits of essential oils. Regular use can help maintain mental and emotional balance over time.

5. Listen to Your Body: Pay attention to how your body and mind respond to different oils. Adjust your blends and usage as needed to ensure they are providing the desired effects.

Chronic Conditions and Long-term Use of Essential Oils

Essential oils can provide ongoing support for managing chronic conditions and improving quality of life. This chapter explores how essential oils can be used to alleviate symptoms of arthritis, digestive issues, and chronic fatigue syndrome. We'll discuss specific oils, their properties, and how to use them safely over the long term.

Arthritis:

Arthritis is a condition that causes inflammation and pain in the joints. Essential oils with anti-inflammatory and analgesic properties can help manage these symptoms.

Key Oils for Arthritis:
Ginger oil: Known for its warming and

anti-inflammatory properties, ginger oil can help reduce joint pain and stiffness.

Frankincense oil: This oil has powerful anti-inflammatory effects and can help improve mobility and reduce pain.

Lavender oil: Offers analgesic and anti-inflammatory benefits, making it useful for reducing pain and swelling.

Eucalyptus oil: Helps reduce inflammation and provides a cooling effect that can relieve pain.

Arthritis Relief Blend:

- 5 drops Ginger oil
- 4 drops Frankincense oil
- 3 drops Lavender oil
- 2 drops Eucalyptus oil

<u>**How to Use:**</u>

- Massage Oil: Dilute the blend with a carrier oil (such as coconut or jojoba oil) and massage into the affected joints. This can be done 2-3 times a day as needed.

- **Bath Soak**: Add a few drops of the blend to a warm bath to soothe joint pain and reduce inflammation.
- **Compress**: Add a few drops of the blend to a bowl of warm water, soak a cloth in the water, and apply it to the painful joints.

Digestive Issues:

Chronic digestive issues can significantly impact daily life. Essential oils can help soothe the digestive system, reduce inflammation, and alleviate symptoms such as bloating, gas, and indigestion.

Key Oils for Digestive Health:

Peppermint oil: Known for its soothing effects on the digestive tract, peppermint oil can help relieve gas, bloating, and indigestion.

Ginger oil: Helps stimulate digestion and reduce nausea and inflammation.

Fennel oil: Promotes healthy digestion and can help reduce bloating and gas.
Chamomile oil: Offers calming effects that can soothe the digestive tract and reduce inflammation.

Digestive Health Blend:
- 5 drops Peppermint oil
- 4 drops Ginger oil
- 3 drops Fennel oil
- 2 drops Chamomile oil

<u>**How to Use:**</u>
- **Topical Application**: Dilute the blend with a carrier oil and massage it onto the abdomen in a clockwise direction to promote digestion and relieve symptoms.
- **Inhalation**: Add a few drops of the blend to a tissue or cotton ball and inhale deeply before meals to stimulate digestion.
- **Tea**: Although essential oils should be used internally with caution, a drop of peppermint or

ginger oil can be added to a cup of herbal tea to support digestion. Ensure the oil is food-grade and consult with a healthcare provider first.

Chronic Fatigue Syndrome

Chronic fatigue syndrome (CFS) is characterized by extreme fatigue that doesn't improve with rest. Essential oils can help manage symptoms by boosting energy levels, reducing stress, and improving sleep quality.

Key Oils for Chronic Fatigue Syndrome:

Rosemary oil: Known for its stimulating effects, rosemary oil can help improve concentration and reduce mental fatigue.

Peppermint oil: Provides an invigorating effect that can help combat feelings of tiredness and improve alertness.

Lavender oil: Helps promote restful sleep and reduce stress, which can alleviate some symptoms of CFS.

Eucalyptus oil: Offers revitalizing properties that can help improve energy levels and reduce fatigue.

Chronic Fatigue Relief Blend:
- 5 drops Rosemary oil
- 4 drops Peppermint oil
- 3 drops Lavender oil
- 2 drops Eucalyptus oil

How to Use:
- **Diffuser**: Add 5-10 drops of the blend to a diffuser to create an energizing and refreshing environment.
- **Inhalation**: Put a few drops on a tissue or cotton ball and inhale deeply throughout the day to maintain energy levels.

- **Massage Oil:** Dilute the blend with a carrier oil and massage into the back of the neck, temples, and wrists to help reduce fatigue and improve alertness.

Practical Tips for Long-term Use

1. **Rotate Oils**: To prevent sensitization and ensure effectiveness, rotate different essential oils and blends over time.

2. **Monitor Reactions**: Keep track of how your body responds to long-term use of essential oils. If you notice any adverse reactions, discontinue use and consult a healthcare professional.

3. **Consult a Professional**: For chronic conditions, it's important to work with a healthcare provider who can help you integrate essential oils safely and effectively into your treatment plan.

4. **Use High-Quality Oils**: The importance of high quality can never be overemphasized. Ensure you are using pure, therapeutic-grade essential oils for

the best results and to avoid potential side effects from low-quality oils.

5. Stay Informed: Continually educate yourself about essential oils and their uses, as new research and information can provide insights into better managing your chronic conditions.

Chapter 7:

Essential Oils in Everyday Life

Essential oils are incredibly versatile and can be seamlessly integrated into your daily routines, not just for health and wellness, but also for maintaining a clean and pleasant home environment. In this chapter, we will explore how to use essential oils for natural cleaning products, air fresheners, and pest control.

Home and Cleaning

Essential oils can transform your cleaning routine, providing a natural, non-toxic alternative to conventional cleaning products. They offer powerful antiseptic, antibacterial, and antifungal properties that make them perfect for maintaining a clean and healthy home.

Natural Cleaning Products

Commercial cleaning products often contain harsh chemicals that can be harmful to your health and the environment. Essential oils offer a safer alternative without compromising on effectiveness.

Key Oils for Cleaning:

- **Lemon oil:** Known for its powerful antiseptic and antibacterial properties, lemon oil is great for cutting through grease and leaving a fresh, clean scent.
- **Tea Tree oil**: offers strong antimicrobial and antifungal properties, making it ideal for disinfecting surfaces.
- **Lavender oil**: Not only does it have antibacterial properties, but it also adds a calming, pleasant scent to your cleaning products.
- **Eucalyptus:** Known for its germicidal properties, eucalyptus

oil is excellent for disinfecting and deodorizing.

All-Purpose Cleaner Recipe:
- 1 cup distilled water
- 1 cup white vinegar
- 20 drops Lemon oil
- 10 drops Tea Tree oil

<u>How to Use:</u>
1. **Combine Ingredients:** Mix the distilled water, white vinegar, lemon oil, and tea tree oil in a spray bottle.
2. **Shake Well:** Before each use, shake the bottle to ensure the oils are well distributed.
3. **Clean Surfaces:** Spray on countertops, sinks, and other surfaces, then wipe clean with a cloth.

Glass Cleaner Recipe:
- 1 cup distilled water
- 1 cup white vinegar
- 10 drops Lavender oil
- 10 drops Eucalyptus oil

<u>**How to use:**</u>

1. Combine Ingredients: Mix the distilled water, white vinegar, lavender oil, and eucalyptus oil in a spray bottle.

2. Shake Well: Shake the bottle before each use.

3. Clean Glass: Spray onto glass surfaces and wipe with a microfiber cloth for a streak-free shine.

Natural Air Fresheners

Essential oils can be used to create natural air fresheners that not only smell wonderful but also offer various health benefits. Unlike synthetic air fresheners, essential oils do not contain harmful chemicals.

Key oils for Air Fresheners:
- **Lavender oil** offers a calming and relaxing aroma, making it,

perfect for bedrooms and living areas.

- **Peppermint oil:** Provides an invigorating and refreshing scent, making it ideal for bathrooms and kitchens.
- **Orange oil**: known for its uplifting and energizing properties, making it great for any room.
- **Cinnamon oil:** Adds a warm, comforting scent, especially nice during the colder months.

Air Freshener Spray Recipe:
- 1 cup distilled water
- 2 tablespoons witch hazel or vodka (helps the oils disperse)
- 20-30 drops essential oils of your choice (e.g., 10 drops Lavender oil, 10 drops Orange, 5 drops Peppermint oil, 5 drops Cinnamon oil)

How to use:

1. Mix distilled water, witch hazel or vodka, and essential oils in a spray bottle.
2. Shake the bottle before each use.
3. Spray around the room as needed to freshen the air.

Diffusing Essential Oils:

Using a diffuser is another excellent way to freshen the air and enjoy the benefits of essential oils. Simply add water and a few drops of your chosen essential oils to the diffuser, and let it work its magic.

Pest Control

Essential oils can be effective natural repellents against various pests, such as insects and rodents. They offer a safe alternative to chemical pesticides, which can be harmful to humans and pets.

Key Oils for Pest Control:

- **Peppermint oil:** Effective against ants, spiders, and mice.
- **Lemon oil:** Can repel mosquitoes and flies.
- **Lavender oil**: Helps deter moths, fleas, and flies.
- **Tea Tree oil:** Known for its insect-repellent properties.

Ant and Spider Repellent Spray Recipe:
- 1 cup water
- 1 cup white vinegar
- 15 drops Peppermint oil
- 15 drops Tea Tree oil

<u>How to Use:</u>
1. Mix water, white vinegar, peppermint oil, and tea tree oil in a spray bottle.
2. Shake the bottle before each use.
3. Apply it around windows, doors, and other entry points to repel ants and spiders.

Moth Repellent Sachets:
- 10 drops Lavender oil
- 10 drops Cedarwood oil
- Small cotton balls or fabric sachets

How to Use:
1. Mix lavender oil and cedarwood oil.
2. Saturate Cotton Balls: Apply a few drops of the blend to cotton balls or place them in fabric sachets.
3. Place in Closets: Put the sachets in closets, drawers, and storage boxes to repel moths.

Mosquito Repellent Spray Recipe:
- 1 cup water
- 1/2 cup witch hazel
- 20 drops Lemon oil
- 20 drops Eucalyptus oil

How to use:
1. Mix water, witch hazel, lemon oil, and eucalyptus oil in a spray bottle.
2. Shake the bottle before each use.

3. Spray on Skin and Clothing: Apply to skin and clothing to repel mosquitoes, avoiding the face and eyes.

Practical Tips for Using Essential Oils in Everyday Life

1. **Consistency:** Use essential oils regularly for the best results, especially for pest control and maintaining a fresh-smelling home.

2. **Safety First:** Always dilute essential oils properly before applying them to surfaces or your skin. Essential oils are potent and can cause irritation if used undiluted.

3. **Test First:** Before using a new essential oil blend on surfaces, test it on a small, inconspicuous area to ensure it doesn't cause any damage or discoloration.

4. **Proper Storage:** Store essential oils and homemade products in dark, glass containers away from direct sunlight to

preserve their potency and extend their shelf life.

5. **Eco-Friendly:** Using essential oils for cleaning and pest control is not only good for your health but also for the environment. They reduce the need for harsh chemicals and minimize waste.

Beauty and Personal Care

Essential oils can play a significant role in enhancing your beauty and personal care routine. They offer natural solutions for skincare, hair care, and overall body care, free from the synthetic chemicals found in many commercial products. This section will cover DIY skincare recipes, hair care treatments, and bath and body products.

DIY Skincare Recipes

Using essential oils in skincare can help address various skin issues, from dryness to acne, thanks to their anti-inflammatory, antibacterial, and soothing properties.

Key Oils for Skincare:

- **Lavender oil:** Calming and soothing, ideal for sensitive and irritated skin.
- **Tea Tree oil:** Antibacterial and antifungal, great for acne-prone skin.
- **Frankincense oil:** Anti-aging properties that can help reduce the appearance of wrinkles and scars.
- **Geranium oil:** Balances oil production and improves overall skin health.

Simple Face Serum Recipe:

- 1 tablespoon jojoba oil (carrier oil)
- 3 drops Frankincense oil
- 3 drops Lavender oil

- 2 drops Geranium oil

<u>How to Use:</u>
1. Mix the oils in a small glass bottle with a dropper.
2. Use a few drops of the serum on your face after cleansing, morning and night.

Acne Spot Treatment:
- 1 tablespoon aloe vera gel
- 2 drops Tea Tree oil
- 1 drop Lavender oil

<u>How to Use:</u>
1. Combine the aloe vera gel and essential oils in a small container.
2. Dab a small amount onto blemishes as needed.

Moisturizing Body Butter:
- 1/2 cup shea butter
- 1/4 cup coconut oil
- 10 drops Lavender oil
- 5 drops Frankincense oil

<u>**How to Use:**</u>

1. **Melt Ingredients**: Gently melt the shea butter and coconut oil together.
2. Mix and Cool: Remove from heat, add essential oils, and let it cool slightly.
3. **Whip:** Use a mixer to whip the mixture until fluffy. Store in a glass jar and use as a body moisturizer.

Hair Care Treatments

Essential oils can be highly beneficial for hair health, promoting growth, adding shine, and addressing scalp issues.

Key Oils for Hair Care:

- **Rosemary oil:** Stimulates hair growth and improves scalp health.
- **Lavender oil:** Soothes the scalp and can help with dandruff.
- **Peppermint oil:** Invigorates the scalp and promotes hair growth.
- **Tea Tree oil:** helps with dandruff and keeps the scalp clean.

Hair Growth Serum:
- 2 tablespoons jojoba oil (carrier oil)
- 5 drops Rosemary oil
- 5 drops Peppermint oil

How to Use:
1.Mix the oils in a small glass bottle.
2. Massage a few drops into your scalp before bed. Leave it on overnight and wash your hair in the morning.

Dandruff Treatment:
- 2 tablespoons coconut oil
- 5 drops Tea Tree oil
- 5 drops Lavender oil

How to Use:
1. Mix the coconut oil and essential oils.
2. Massage into your scalp and leave for at least 30 minutes before washing your hair.

Bath and Body Products

With essential oils that can calm, stimulate, or relax your body and mind, you can completely change the experience of taking a bath.

Relaxing Bath Soak:
- 1 cup Epsom salt
- 1/2 cup baking soda
- 10 drops Lavender oil
- 5 drops Ylang-Ylang oil

How to Use:
1. Combine Epsom salt, baking soda, and essential oils in a jar.
2. Add a few tablespoons to a warm bath and soak for 20-30 minutes.

Refreshing Body Scrub:
- 1 cup sugar
- 1/2 cup coconut oil
- 10 drops Lemon oil
- 5 drops Peppermint oil

<u>**How to Use:**</u>

1. Mix sugar and coconut oil, then add essential oils.

2. Scrub: Use in the shower to exfoliate and invigorate your skin.

Cooking and Food Preservation

Essential oils can also be used in the kitchen to flavor food and help with food preservation. They offer a concentrated source of flavor and have antimicrobial properties that can enhance food safety.

Flavoring Food

Using essential oils in cooking can add a burst of flavor, but it's important to use them sparingly due to their potency.

Key Oils for Cooking:

- Lemon oil: Adds a bright, citrusy flavor to dishes.

- **Peppermint oil:** enhances desserts and beverages with a refreshing taste.
- **Basil oil:** great for adding a herbal note to savory dishes.
- **Lavender oil:** Can be used in baking for a subtle floral flavor.

Lemon Drizzle Cake:

- 1 drop Lemon oil (ensure it's food-grade)
- 1 cup sugar
- 1/2 cup butter
- 2 eggs
- 1 1/2 cups flour
- 1/2 cup milk
- 1 teaspoon baking powder

How to Use:

1. **Mix Wet Ingredients**: Cream together butter and sugar, then add eggs and Lemon oil.
2. **Add dry ingredients:** Mix in flour and baking powder, then add milk.

3. Bake: Pour into a greased pan and bake at 350°F for 30-40 minutes.

Peppermint Hot Chocolate:
- 1 drop Peppermint oil (ensure it's food-grade)
- 2 cups milk
- 1/4 cup cocoa powder
- 1/4 cup sugar

How to Use:

1. Heat Milk: Warm the milk in a saucepan.
2. Add Cocoa and Sugar: Whisk in cocoa powder and sugar until dissolved.
3. Add Peppermint: Stir in the drop of Peppermint oil before serving.

Food Safety and Preservation

Essential oils can help preserve food by inhibiting the growth of bacteria and mold. They should be used with care and in appropriate amounts.

Key Oils for Food Preservation:

- **Clove oil:** Known for its strong antimicrobial properties.
- **Lemon oil:** Helps inhibit the growth of bacteria.
- **Oregano oil:** Offers powerful antibacterial effects.
- **Cinnamon oil:** Can prevent mold growth and has antimicrobial benefits.

Recipe for Preserving Fresh Produce:

- 1 cup water
- 10 drops Lemon oil
- 10 drops Oregano oil

<u>**How to Use:**</u>

1. Mix Ingredients: Combine water and essential oils in a spray bottle.
2. Spray Produce: Lightly spray on fresh produce before storing to extend shelf life and reduce spoilage.

Extending Shelf Life of Baked Foods:

- Add 1-2 drops of Cinnamon or Clove oil to the dough or batter to inhibit mold growth and extend freshness.

Practical Tips for Using Essential Oils in Beauty and Food

1. **Use Sparingly:** Essential oils are very potent, so a little goes a long way, especially in cooking.
2. **Quality Matters:** Ensure you are using food-grade essential oils when incorporating them into recipes.
3. **Patch Test:** Always perform a patch test when using essential oils in skincare to check for allergic reactions.
4. **Proper Storage:** Store essential oils and DIY products in dark, glass containers away from direct sunlight to maintain their potency.
5. **Educate Yourself:** Continually learn about the properties and safe uses

of essential oils to maximize their benefits while minimizing risks.

Chapter 8:

Purchasing and Storing Essential Oils

When it comes to essential oils, choosing the right ones and storing them properly are essential steps to ensure their effectiveness and longevity. In this chapter, we'll discuss where to buy essential oils, what to look for on labels, and how to store them correctly to preserve their quality.

Where to Buy

Essential oils are available from various sources, but it's essential to purchase them from reputable brands and suppliers to ensure their quality and purity.

Reputable Brands and Suppliers:
- **Health Food Stores:** Many health food stores carry a selection

of essential oils from trusted brands.

- **Online Retailers:** Websites like Amazon, and the official websites of reputable essential oil companies offer a wide range of options.
- **Specialty Stores:** Some stores specialize in aromatherapy and natural products and may offer a curated selection of high-quality essential oils.

What to Look for on Labels:

1. **Botanical Name:** Each essential oil should list its botanical name to ensure you're getting the correct plant species.

2. **Purity:** Look for labels indicating that the oil is 100% pure and free from additives or synthetic ingredients.

3. **Extraction Method:** The label should specify how the oil was extracted (e.g., steam distillation, cold-pressing).

4. **Country of Origin:** Knowing where the plant was grown can give you insight into its quality.

5. **Certifications:** Some oils may be certified organic or have other quality certifications.

Storing Your Oils

Proper storage is crucial for maintaining the potency and shelf life of essential oils. Follow these guidelines to ensure your oils stay fresh and effective.

Shelf Life:
- Essential oils have varying shelf lives depending on the oil and its constituents. Generally, most oils have a shelf life of 1-3 years when stored properly.
- Citrus oils tend to have a shorter shelf life due to their high volatility, while oils with higher concentrations of sesquiterpenes

(like sandalwood and patchouli) can last longer.

Proper Storage Conditions:

1. Dark Glass Bottles: Essential oils should be stored in dark glass bottles to protect them from light, which can degrade their quality.

2. Cool, Dark Place: Store oils in a cool, dark place away from direct sunlight and heat sources, such as radiators or stoves.

3. Airtight Containers: Ensure the bottles are tightly sealed to prevent oxidation, which can cause oils to degrade more quickly.

4. Avoid Extreme Temperatures: Fluctuations in temperature can affect the consistency and potency of essential oils, so avoid storing them in areas prone to temperature changes, such as bathrooms or near windows.

5. Keep Away from Children and Pets: Essential oils are potent and can be harmful if ingested. Store them out of reach of children and pets.

Practical Tips for Purchasing and Storing Essential Oils

1. Do Your Research: Take the time to research brands and suppliers to ensure you're purchasing high-quality oils.

2. Read Reviews: Check online reviews and customer feedback to learn about others' experiences with specific oils and brands.

3. Start Small: When trying a new brand or oil, start with a small quantity to test its quality and effectiveness.

4. Keep Track of Expiry Dates: Label your oils with the purchase date and expiration date to track their shelf life.

5. Rotate Your Stock: Use older oils first to ensure you're always using the freshest products.

Recognizing Quality Essential Oils

Ensuring the quality of essential oils is crucial for their effectiveness and safety. In this section, we'll discuss how to recognize quality oils, including certifications and purity tests, and how to avoid adulterated products.

Certifications and Purity Tests

Certifications: Look for essential oils that have undergone third-party testing and have received certifications from reputable organizations. Some common certifications include:

- **Certified Organic:** Indicates that the plants used to produce the oil were grown without synthetic pesticides or fertilizers.
- **GC/MS Testing:** Gas Chromatography/Mass Spectrometry (GC/MS) is a common method used to analyze

the chemical composition of essential oils and ensure their purity.

- **ISO Certification:** International Organization for Standardization (ISO) certification verifies that the oil meets specific quality and safety standards.

Purity Tests: Reputable essential oil companies conduct purity tests to ensure their products are free from contaminants and adulterants. These tests may include:

- **Gas Chromatography (GC):** Separates and analyzes the individual components of the oil to identify any impurities or synthetic additives.

- **Mass Spectrometry (MS):** Determines the molecular structure of the oil's components, providing further insight into its purity and quality.

- **Organoleptic Testing:** Involves evaluating the oil's aroma, color, and consistency to detect any abnormalities or signs of contamination.

Avoiding Adulterated Products

Adulteration occurs when inferior or synthetic substances are added to essential oils to reduce costs or enhance fragrance. To avoid purchasing adulterated products, consider the following:

- **Research Brands:** Choose reputable brands with a track record of transparency and quality. Look for companies that prioritize sourcing high-quality botanicals and conducting rigorous testing.
- **Check Labels:** Read the label carefully to ensure it contains only the botanical name of the oil and

doesn't include any additional ingredients or fillers.

- **Beware of Unrealistically Low Prices:** Quality essential oils require a significant amount of plant material and extraction processes, so extremely low prices may indicate inferior quality or adulteration.

- **Trust Your Senses:** Pay attention to the aroma, color, and consistency of the oil. While synthetic additives may mimic the fragrance of natural oils, they often lack the complexity and depth of true essential oils.

Practical Tips for Recognizing Quality

1. Educate Yourself: Learn about the botanical origins, extraction methods, and quality standards for essential oils to make informed purchasing decisions.

2. Ask Questions: Don't hesitate to reach out to the manufacturer or supplier with questions about their sourcing, testing, and production processes.

3. Read Reviews: Check online reviews and testimonials from other customers to gauge the quality and reputation of the brand.

4. Start Small: When trying a new brand or oil, purchase a small quantity to test its quality and effectiveness before committing to larger quantities.

5. Trust Your Intuition: If something seems too good to be true or doesn't feel right, trust your instincts and consider exploring other options.

Chapter 9:

The Science Behind Essential Oils

Understanding the science behind essential oils can deepen your appreciation for their benefits and guide you in using them more effectively. This chapter explores the phytochemistry of essential oils, the therapeutic actions of their active compounds, current research and evidence, and future trends in the field.

Phytochemistry of Essential Oils

Phytochemistry refers to the study of the chemicals derived from plants. Essential oils are complex mixtures of volatile compounds, which are responsible for their fragrance and therapeutic properties.

Active Compounds:

Terpenes: These are the largest group of natural compounds found in essential oils. They include monoterpenes (like limonene in citrus oils) and sesquiterpenes (like chamazulene in chamomile oil), known for their anti-inflammatory, antiviral, and antiseptic properties.

Phenols: Compounds like eugenol in clove oil and thymol in thyme oil are powerful antioxidants and have strong antimicrobial properties.

Aldehydes: Citral in lemongrass oil and cinnamaldehyde in cinnamon oil are known for their calming effects and antimicrobial actions.

Ketones: Compounds like menthone in peppermint oil have mucolytic properties, which help in breaking down mucus.

Esters: Linalyl acetate in lavender oil and geranyl acetate in bergamot oil are soothing and anti-inflammatory.

Oxides: 1,8-cineole in eucalyptus oil has expectorant and anti-inflammatory properties.

Therapeutic Actions:
The therapeutic actions of essential oils are largely due to their active compounds, which can have a range of effects on the body:

Antimicrobial: Many essential oils, such as tea tree and oregano, have strong antimicrobial properties, making them effective against bacteria, viruses, and fungi.

Anti-inflammatory: Oils like frankincense and chamomile can reduce inflammation and promote healing.

Antioxidant: Essential oils such as clove and rosemary are rich in antioxidants, which can help protect the body from oxidative stress.

Sedative: Lavender and ylang-ylang oils are known for their calming and sedative effects, helping to reduce stress and promote sleep.

Stimulant: Peppermint and rosemary oils can invigorate the mind and body, enhancing concentration and energy.

Research and Evidence

Current Studies:
The scientific community has shown growing interest in essential oils, leading to numerous studies that investigate their efficacy and safety. Some key areas of research include:

- **Antimicrobial Properties:** Studies have confirmed the effectiveness of essential oils like tea tree and oregano in combating various pathogens.
- **Anti-inflammatory Effects:** Research has demonstrated that oils such as frankincense and

chamomile can significantly reduce inflammation.

- **Mental Health Benefits:** Essential oils like lavender and bergamot have been shown to reduce anxiety and improve mood in clinical trials.
- **Pain Management:** Peppermint and eucalyptus oils have been studied for their analgesic and muscle-relaxant properties.

Efficacy and Limitations:

While there is substantial evidence supporting the benefits of essential oils, it's important to recognize their limitations:

- **Variability in Quality:** The efficacy of essential oils can vary greatly depending on their quality, purity, and method of use.
- **Lack of Standardization:** There is no standardized dosage or application method for essential

oils, making it challenging to compare studies and results.

- **Potential Side Effects:** Some individuals may experience allergic reactions or sensitivities to certain oils, and incorrect use can lead to adverse effects.

Future of Essential Oils

Emerging Trends:
As interest in natural health products grows, several trends are emerging in the field of essential oils:

- **Personalized Aromatherapy:** Advances in technology are making it possible to tailor essential oil blends to individual needs and preferences.
- **Sustainability:** There is a growing focus on the sustainable and ethical sourcing of essential oils to protect plant species and ecosystems.

- **Integrative Medicine:** Essential oils are increasingly being incorporated into mainstream healthcare practices, such as in hospitals and wellness centers.

Technological Advancements:

Technological advancements are enhancing the extraction, analysis, and application of essential oils:

- **Improved Extraction Methods:** Techniques like supercritical CO_2 extraction are being used to obtain purer and more potent essential oils.
- **Enhanced Delivery Systems:** New methods, such as nanoemulsions and encapsulation, are being developed to improve the absorption and effectiveness of essential oils.
- **Smart Diffusers:** These devices can be programmed to release essential oils at specific times and

concentrations, optimizing their benefits.

The science behind essential oils is a fascinating blend of chemistry and biology, revealing the complex interactions between plant compounds and the human body. Through ongoing research, we are gaining a deeper understanding of their therapeutic potential and limitations. As technology and trends evolve, the future of essential oils looks promising, with more personalized and effective applications on the horizon. Embracing this knowledge can enhance your use of essential oils, allowing you to harness their full potential safely and effectively.

CONCLUSION

As we wrap up our journey through the world of essential oils, let's take a moment to recap key points, offer some encouragement for further exploration, and provide a few final tips and reminders to help you on your path.

Recap of Key Points

Understanding Essential Oils: Essential oils are highly concentrated plant extracts with unique properties. They have a rich history and diverse uses, ranging from physical and mental health benefits to applications in beauty, cleaning, and cooking.

Extraction Methods: Various methods, such as steam distillation and cold pressing, are used to extract essential oils, each impacting the oil's quality and properties.

Benefits and Uses: Essential oils can support physical health by alleviating common ailments, boosting the immune system, and promoting respiratory health. They also offer mental and emotional benefits, including stress relief, mood enhancement, and improved cognitive function.

Safety Guidelines: Proper dilution, patch testing, and safe storage are crucial for using essential oils safely. Specific considerations should be made for pregnant and breastfeeding women, children, and pets.

Blending and Application: Understanding how to create your own blends and use essential oils in various ways, such as through diffusers, topical applications, and even cooking, can maximize their benefits.

Quality and Purity: Knowing how to identify high-quality essential oils through certifications, purity tests, and careful brand selection ensures you get the best out of your oils.

Science and Future Trends: The ongoing research into essential oils' efficacy and safety continues to unveil new uses and applications, promising a bright future for this ancient practice.

Encouragement for Further Exploration

Your journey with essential oils is just beginning. The more you learn and experiment, the more you'll discover about these powerful natural products. Here are a few ways to deepen your exploration:

Read More: Dive into books, articles, and research papers on aromatherapy and essential oils. There's a wealth of knowledge out there.

Take Classes: Look for workshops or online courses that can provide hands-on learning and expert insights.

Join Communities: Engage with online forums, social media groups, or local clubs focused on essential oils. Sharing experiences and tips with others can be incredibly enriching.

Experiment: Don't be afraid to try new blends and applications. Keep a journal of your experiences, noting what works best for you and your loved ones.

In conclusion, essential oils are a wonderful addition to your wellness toolkit, offering a myriad of benefits for the body, mind, and home. By understanding their properties, uses, and safety guidelines, you can confidently explore the world of aromatherapy and harness the power of these natural wonders. Remember to stay curious, prioritize safety, and enjoy the journey.

APPENDICES

To help you navigate and utilize essential oils more effectively, we've included a comprehensive glossary of terms and conversion charts. These appendices provide definitions of key terms and practical measurements to assist you in your essential oil journey.

Glossary of Terms

Absorption: The process by which essential oils enter the body through the skin or mucous membranes.

Adulteration: The practice of adding synthetic substances or inferior oils to essential oils to dilute or mimic their properties.

Aldehydes: Organic compounds found in some essential oils, known for their calming and antimicrobial properties.

Antimicrobial: A property of essential oils that allows them to kill or inhibit the growth of microorganisms, including bacteria, viruses, and fungi.

Antioxidant: Compounds that protect the body from oxidative stress by neutralizing free radicals.

Aromatherapy: The therapeutic use of essential oils to promote physical, emotional, and mental well-being.

Base Note: The longest-lasting fragrance component of an essential oil blend, which provides depth and stability.

Botanical Name: The scientific name of a plant, used to precisely identify the species and ensure the correct essential oil is being used.

Carrier Oil: A vegetable oil used to dilute essential oils for safe topical application.

Chemotype: The chemical composition of a plant that can vary within the same species, resulting in different therapeutic properties.

Cold Pressing: A method of extracting essential oils from citrus fruits by pressing the rinds to release the oil.

Distillation: A common method of extracting essential oils using steam to separate the oil from the plant material.

Esters: Organic compounds in essential oils known for their soothing and anti-inflammatory properties.

GC/MS Testing: Gas Chromatography/Mass Spectrometry, a testing method used to analyze the chemical composition and purity of essential oils.

Hydrosol: The water-based byproduct of steam distillation, containing small amounts of essential oil and water-soluble plant compounds.

Middle Note: The heart of an essential oil blend that bridges the top and base notes, often with balancing and harmonizing properties.

Monoterpenes: A class of terpenes commonly found in essential oils, known for their antimicrobial and anti-inflammatory effects.

Organoleptic Testing: The evaluation of essential oils based on sensory characteristics such as smell, color, and texture.

Oxides: Compounds in essential oils, like 1,8-cineole, known for their expectorant and anti-inflammatory properties.

Patch Test: A method to check for skin sensitivity to essential oils by applying a diluted drop to a small area of skin and observing for any reaction.

Phenols: Powerful compounds in essential oils with strong antimicrobial and antioxidant properties.

Phytochemistry: The study of the chemical compounds produced by plants, including those found in essential oils.

Purity: The quality of an essential oil being free from additives, synthetic substances, or contaminants.

Sesquiterpenes: Heavier, more complex terpenes in essential oils that often provide grounding and calming effects.

Steam Distillation: A method of extracting essential oils using steam to separate the oil from the plant material.

Synergy: The enhanced effect that occurs when different essential oils are blended together, creating a combination that is more effective than the individual oils.

Terpenes: The primary constituents of essential oils, responsible for their aroma and therapeutic properties.

Top Note: The initial, most volatile scent component of an essential oil blend that evaporates quickly.

Volatility: The tendency of essential oils to evaporate at room temperature, contributing to their aroma and potency.

Conversion Charts

Proper measurement is crucial when working with essential oils. Here are some handy conversion charts to help you accurately dilute and blend your oils.

Volume Conversions:
- 1 milliliter (ml) = 20 drops (approx.)
- 1 teaspoon (tsp) = 5 ml = 100 drops
- 1 tablespoon (tbsp) = 15 ml = 300 drops
- 1 fluid ounce (oz) = 30 ml = 600 drops

Dilution Ratios:
To safely use essential oils, they need to be diluted with a carrier oil. Here are some common dilution ratios for different purposes:

General Dilution for Adults:
- 1% dilution: 1 drop of essential oil per teaspoon of carrier oil
- 2% dilution: 2 drops of essential oil per teaspoon of carrier oil
- 3% dilution: 3 drops of essential oil per teaspoon of carrier oil

For Children (Ages 2-12):
- 1% dilution: 1 drop of essential oil per teaspoon of carrier oil

For Infants (Under 2 Years):
- 0.25%-0.5% dilution: 1 drop of essential oil per 4 teaspoons of carrier oil

For Sensitive Skin or Elderly:
- 1% dilution: 1 drop of essential oil per teaspoon of carrier oil

Common Blending Measurements:
When creating your own blends, it's helpful to use consistent measurements.

Here are some basic conversions for blending:

Essential Oil Blending:
- 1% dilution: 6 drops of essential oil per ounce of carrier oil
- 2% dilution: 12 drops of essential oil per ounce of carrier oil
- 3% dilution: 18 drops of essential oil per ounce of carrier oil
- 5% dilution: 30 drops of essential oil per ounce of carrier oil
- 10% dilution: 60 drops of essential oil per ounce of carrier oil

Quick Reference for Drop-to-Volume Conversions:
- 10 drops = 0.5 ml
- 20 drops = 1 ml
- 50 drops = 2.5 ml
- 100 drops = 5 ml

Dilution Guidelines, Safety Checklist, and Recipes and Blending Sheets

To ensure the safe and effective use of essential oils, it's crucial to understand proper dilution guidelines, follow a comprehensive safety checklist, and use recipes and blending sheets. This section will provide detailed information on these topics to help you get the most out of your essential oils.

Dilution Guidelines

Essential oils are highly concentrated and should be diluted before topical application to prevent skin irritation and sensitization. Here are some guidelines for diluting essential oils with a carrier oil:

General Dilution Ratios:

- **1% Dilution:** Ideal for facial applications, sensitive skin, and children. Use 1 drop of essential oil per teaspoon (5 ml) of carrier oil.

- **2% Dilution:** Suitable for daily body care products, such as lotions and creams. Use 2 drops of essential oil per teaspoon (5 ml) of carrier oil.
- **3% Dilution:** For specific treatments, such as massage oils for sore muscles. Use 3 drops of essential oil per teaspoon (5 ml) of carrier oil.
- **5% Dilution:** For acute issues like muscle pain or respiratory problems, but only for short-term use. Use 5 drops of essential oil per teaspoon (5 ml) of carrier oil.
- **10% Dilution:** For small areas of concern, like a dab on a pimple or insect bite. Use 10 drops of essential oil per teaspoon (5 ml) of carrier oil.

Specific Dilution Guidelines:

- **Infants (Under 2 Years):** Use a 0.25%-0.5% dilution. This equates to 1 drop of essential oil per 4 teaspoons (20 ml) of carrier oil.

- **Children (Ages 2-12):** Use a 1% dilution, which is 1 drop of essential oil per teaspoon (5 ml) of carrier oil.

- **Pregnant Women:** Use a 1% dilution to ensure safety. Consult a healthcare provider before use.

- **Elderly or Those with Sensitive Skin:** Use a 1% dilution to avoid irritation.

Safety Checklist

When using essential oils, safety should always be a top priority. Here is a comprehensive checklist to ensure safe practice:

1. Patch Test: Always perform a patch test before using a new essential oil.

Apply a small amount of diluted oil to a patch of skin and wait 24 hours to check for any reaction.

2. Dilution: Always dilute essential oils before applying them to the skin. Refer to the dilution guidelines to determine the appropriate ratio.

3. Avoid Sensitive Areas: Do not apply essential oils to sensitive areas such as the eyes, ears, mucous membranes, or broken skin.

4. Use High-Quality Oils: Choose 100% pure, high-quality essential oils from reputable sources to avoid synthetic additives and contaminants.

5. Storage: Store essential oils in dark glass bottles in a cool, dark place, out of reach of children and pets.

6. Read Labels: Pay attention to any warnings or contraindications on the oil's label.

7. Consult a Professional: If you are pregnant, nursing, have a medical condition, or are taking medications, consult a healthcare provider before using essential oils.

8. Educate Yourself: Learn about each essential oil's properties and potential side effects before use.

9. Internal Use: Be cautious with internal use of essential oils. Consult a healthcare professional before ingesting any essential oil.

10. Sun Sensitivity: Some essential oils, particularly citrus oils, can cause photosensitivity. Avoid sun exposure after applying these oils to the skin or use sunscreen when going outside on hot days.

Recipes and Blending Sheets

Having some go-to recipes and blending sheets can make using essential oils more straightforward and enjoyable. Here are a few recipes for common uses and a basic blending sheet to get you started.

<u>**Common Recipes:**</u>

Relaxing Massage Oil:
- 2 tablespoons (30 ml) of sweet almond oil (carrier oil)
- 3 drops of lavender essential oil
- 2 drops of chamomile essential oil
- 1 drop of frankincense essential oil

Combine all ingredients in a dark glass bottle and shake well. Use for a soothing massage.

Energizing Room Spray:
- 1/2 cup (120 ml) of distilled water
- 1 tablespoon (15 ml) of witch hazel
- 10 drops of peppermint essential oil
- 10 drops of lemon essential oil

Mix all ingredients in a spray bottle and shake well before each use. Spray around the room for an invigorating atmosphere.

Calming Bath Soak:

- 1 cup (240 ml) of Epsom salts
- 1 tablespoon (15 ml) of carrier oil (such as jojoba or coconut oil)
- 5 drops of lavender essential oil
- 3 drops of ylang-ylang essential oil

Combine all ingredients in a bowl and mix well. Add to a warm bath and soak for 20 minutes to relax.

Basic Blending Sheet:

Blending Notes:
- **Top Notes:** Evaporate quickly, provide the initial impression (e.g., citrus oils like lemon, grapefruit).
- **Middle Notes:** Provide the body of the blend, last longer than top notes (e.g., lavender, geranium).
- **Base Notes:** Last the longest, provide depth and grounding (e.g., sandalwood, patchouli).

Blending Ratios:
- For a balanced blend, aim for a ratio of 30% top notes, 50% middle notes, and 20% base notes.

Example Blend for Stress Relief:
- Top Note: 3 drops of bergamot
- Middle Note: 5 drops of lavender
- Base Note: 2 drops of frankincense

Record your blends, noting the number of drops and the essential oils used. This helps you recreate successful blends and refine your techniques.

Dilution guidelines, safety checklists, and well-crafted recipes are essential tools for safely and effectively using essential oils. By following these guidelines, you can enjoy the numerous benefits of essential oils while minimizing the risk of adverse reactions. Keep a record of your blends and continue learning to enhance your aromatherapy practices.

www.ingramcontent.com/pod-product-compliance
Lightning Source LLC
Chambersburg PA
CBHW012255240726
48656CB00007B/2390